THE HEALING POWER
OF OUR LOVE

THE HEALING POWER OF OUR LOVE

James A. Ryan, M.D., J.D.

The torch is a symbol of light, enlightenment, and inspiration. My book sheds some new light on the soul as the inspirational source of our loving and healing energies.

iUniverse, Inc.
New York Bloomington

THE HEALING POWER OF OUR LOVE

iUniverse books may be ordered through booksellers or by contacting:

iUniverse
1663 Liberty Drive
Bloomington, IN 47403
www.iuniverse.com
1-800-Authors (1-800-288-4677)

Because of the dynamic nature of the Internet, any Web addresses or links contained in this book may have changed since publication and may no longer be valid.

The views expressed in this work are solely those of the author and do not necessarily reflect the views of the publisher, and the publisher hereby disclaims any responsibility for them.

ISBN: 978-1-4401-1486-1 (pbk)
ISBN: 978-1-4401-1487-8 (ebk)

Printed in the United States of America

Contents

Acknowledgments

I want to express my gratitude to a number of people who have made this book possible. First and foremost is my wife Priscilla who lovingly endured my preoccupation with its writing on many vacations and weekends. The same is true for our three children, Maureen, Jimmy and Patrick. My first editor was Mr. Tom Congdon, the literary seer of Nantucket, who imparted a much-needed professional touch. He emphasized that I was writing for people of above average intelligence, and so I selected five good friends to be the first readers. Mrs. Jean Joyce Comstock, with a Master's Degree in Psychiatric Nursing, is a healer who has always been there for friends in their hour of need. Her inner warmth as a student nurse at Georgetown caught my eye and helped me to learn about the healing quality of this personal asset. Dr. Francis Barnes, perhaps the most highly regarded psychiatrist in Washington, had been one of my teachers. He encouraged me to bring out the humane elements in psychiatric practice. Mrs. Joan Cormack, and her husband Tom were long-time friends who also made many valuable suggestions. Mrs. Pat Normile looked at it last and rearranged the first chapter. Three other professional editors, and writers with helpful advice were Mrs. Maureen Bowen of Manhattan, Mrs. Angela Cox of Pelham, New York, and columnist Colman McCarthy of D.C., whose wife Mav is also a dear friend.

Inspirational sermons are a wonderful tonic for the soul. Some of the very finest have been delivered by Monsignors Louis Quinn, Thomas Duffy, John Enzler, William English, Peter Vaghi, and Fathers William Byrons, S.J., Al Novotny, S.J. and James Greenfield, O.S.

My wife and I are especially indebted to the Sisters of the Visitation Convent for sharing their rich spirituality. Mother Philomena and Sisters DeSales and Berchmans have preserved the Visitation tradition well.

I salute the Order of Malta and some of the many who have made our pilgrimages to Lourdes such a Blessing. Our leader, Adm. Bill Callaghan, and his wife Betty, Shep and Kathryn Abell, Bill and Mary Noel Page, Jim and Rosemary Belson, John Dorment, Carroll and Rosemary Carter, Mike Miskovsky, and the medical committee, all with spouses: Jim Foster, Yacek Mostwin, Dan Finkelstein, Patty McCarthy, Don Joyce, Joe Swift, Dick Perry, and John Harvey.

I look forward to surprising my three living siblings, Rich and Terry Ryan, and my sister, Sr. Sarah Ryan, with copies of the book.

Last but not least, I want to thank Mr. Steve Goth, without whose electronic wizardry there would be no book.

Preface

In an era of alarm about human nature, "The Healing Power Of Our Love" takes a decidedly upbeat stance on the human condition. My optimism is based on the improvements in health I have seen when doctors share their inner personal warmth with patients.

I trained on The Harvard Psychiatric Service at Boston's Beth Israel Hospital under one of Freud's most well known pupils, Dr.Grete Bibring. She taught her Fellows that their first responsibility was to be a caring physician, and assigned us to make daily visits with seriously ill medical and surgical patients. Many of them were able to live much longer than expected as a result of this extra dosage of care. Dr. Bibring also told us that Freud's greatest disappointment had been his failure to solve the mystery of schizophrenia. She suggested I work on this problem by citing Freud's promise that its solution would yield a new perspective on human nature.

As Chief Psychiatrist at the District of Columbia General Hospital I watched our staff overcome the deep withdrawal and delusional thinking of schizophrenics by reaching a "warming point" with them on admission. Patients then became able to share caring feelings with one another, and to work together to reason their way out of their delusions. We had discovered a powerful healing love drive present in the inner warmth of each and every one of us. Our hospital became the only one of its kind in the world able to discard the use of restraints and unlock all its doors, allowing our patients free access to the outside world. Most of them were able to go home in a few days. Over two years of operating this way we witnessed the almost miraculous healing of several thousand acutely ill schizophrenics. We had solved the mystery of schizophrenia and come upon a profound secret of human nature. A bond of caring energies joins us with one another, in a linkage that must remain intact for rationality to exist. Man is primarily a caring animal whose rationality depends on being able to share inner warmth with others.

The book traces the operation of shared inner warmth through clinical vignettes of the successful treatment of schizophrenia, drug-resistant suicidal depressions, borderline personality disorders, senility and organic illnesses. Twentieth Century psychiatry was governed by a three dimensional model of the mind, consisting of the ego, superego and id. My book offers new medical evidence to support a fourth dimension, more powerful by far than the other three. It is the human soul where both God and man reside and interact to generate the healing power of shared inner warmth. The many and vital psychological functions of the soul are discussed in the last two chapters.

1

About that law degree

Over the years a number of people have asked me how I came to have degrees in both law and medicine. When I was in my third year in high school the English teacher asked us to write an essay on the kind of career we were contemplating. I had been reading a book about the diplomatic service and was impressed with the glamour and intrigue of their work, so I made it my choice. Classmates thought it was a pretty good call and voted me the second most likely to succeed, just behind an already well to do young man who planned to be a financier on Wall Street. Of course neither of us made it there, and by senior year I was sure that I would become a doctor or lawyer, but certainly not both.

World War Two was still on and the choice had to be made quickly before starting in college a month after graduation. I already had my favorite job of all time during that month as a lifeguard at Rockaway Beach. Perched in the splendid isolation of the lifeguard chair, high above the sand in the realm of the birds, I asked myself "What do you really want to be?" My high school, Regis High in New York, had a marvelous esprit de corps that encouraged us to aim high in life. I knew that a number of our alumni had become high-powered lawyers and were earning handsome salaries. I was sure that I could join in their success. But then I thought what I'd really like to do is to help other people, and this could be done much better as a doctor. The immediate question was what kind of doctor? I didn't want to be a surgeon or obstetrician and had some misgivings about being a GP. I had read somewhere that the World War was producing a great need for more doctors to help the many servicemen who had serious posttraumatic stress disorders. The psychiatrists needed to meet this task would be younger men who could think differently from the many that only knew how to work in the state hospital systems. They would have to be more psychologically minded and even well versed in the writings of Sigmund Freud. It was frankly exciting for me to think about taking on such a challenge so I decided to become a pre-med student at Fordham College. I also made up my mind to join the Marine Corps while I was still seventeen, immediately after the first year in college. Love of our country was a powerful motivating force in those days. Most of us felt it was a special privilege to serve in the armed forces, and my love of the Marine Corps remains strong to this day. I was probably the only marine who carried a chemistry textbook in the top of his seabag for study in free moments.

In my junior year in medical school I encountered my first serious doubts about the wisdom of becoming a psychiatrist. A month spent in St. Elizabeth's Hospital, the "state hospital" for D.C., was a daily nightmare. I met my very first patient, my "case study", on a locked ward that was filled with pajama clad patients screaming expletives that could be heard outside on the grounds as an eerie babble. My patient sat in their midst, openly and repetitiously masturbating. He was incontinent of urine so that his saturated pajamas produced a pungent urinary stench. I asked a nurse why they didn't do something about these problems and was told he was a hopeless case, because it was his third hospital admission. The only therapeutic measure for the other patients consisted in marching them, one at a time, into a large tiled room where they were greeted with a blast from a fire hose that knocked them off their feet. As they rolled around on the floor they were swatted from top to bottom with the hose until they were barely able to march back to the ward. At the same time I learned from some lawyer friends that the psychiatrists testifying in court were the laughing stock of the legal profession. As I thought these situations over during a medical internship I decided that a psychiatrist with some legal training would be well received in court, and better equipped to deal with abusive situations. I decided to take some classes in Georgetown's Law School just to get my foot into the legal door. I never dreamed of obtaining a law degree, but was impressed with the quality of the teachers there. Edward Bennett Williams in Criminal Law and Professor Walter Jaeger in Contracts were two of the best teachers I had ever had. Content with what I had already learned in law school, I became a Fellow in Psychiatry at Boston's Beth Israel Hospital, and looked forward to a heavy schedule of evening conferences there. I had had no thoughts at all about further legal studies, when I stopped by the Boston College Law School for a social visit with the Dean, Fr. Robert Drinan, S.J. He said that he could see the great value of trying to draw the law and psychiatry closer together, and hoped that I could take at least one course at Boston College. He observed that I had already taken some important first year courses, and asked if I had missed any of the basic courses at Georgetown. I said, "Well, yes, Torts", and he already had the course schedule of B.C.Law in front of him. He asked whether there was any night when I didn't have a conference, and I said "Thursday". Glancing at his protocol, he commented that Torts was already scheduled for Wednesday, and he paused for a moment in deep thought. He finally said, "That's not written in stone, you know", and taking his pen, he scratched the sheet of paper and said, "There. Torts is now scheduled for Thursday, and you'll really like the professor. He's great." I felt like I had just been cast under a spell by a great Shaman, who was determined to chart the course of my life. My two years at Beth Israel allowed for a fruit-ful marriage of law and psychiatry, and one of the teachers at Boston College drafted me to help him conduct a course in Mental Health Law in the Harvard University School of Law.

I can't leave the subject of Fr. Drinan's contribution to my life without mentioning the greatest lesson that he taught. Many readers will remember that his legal career was highlighted by his election to the U.S.House of Representatives, and that he was later told by the Pope that he had to resign from this position. I took great umbrage to this action of the Pope, but Fr. Drinan did not. He surrendered his position quietly and without complaint. What a marvelous lesson in humility for all of us to ponder.

About half-way through law school I decided that I had had enough, and wanted more time in the evenings to spend with my wife. The Dean of Georgetown's Law School, Professor Ken Pye, was a close friend of mine, and in fact I had met my wife at a party in his home. He got together with her, told her that I had already taken all the difficult courses, and would have such an easy schedule of electives that I could go home early every night. And that's how I finally became a doctor with a law degree. It took nine years to get there, but in a later chapter I'll describe how my dual professional life made it possible to reach my most cherished goal as a psychiatrist, the unlocking of D.C.General Hospital. Before going further, I have one other acknowledgment to make. I have learned much more from each and every one of my patients than they have learned from me. My professional growth, in every step of the way, has been fed and fueled by my patients.

2

Inner warmth and the art of medicine

Inner warmth is a quality that goes to the very core of our human nature. It is comprised of the caring, indeed loving energies of each one of us that can be put to good use in healing disturbances like anger, anxiety and depression in others. The supply of loving energies that fuels our inner warmth begins at birth, is powerfully nurtured through eye to eye contact and shared bodily warmth with parents in the first two years, and the exchange of caring energies with other humans over a lifetime. Babies take advantage of the eye to eye route as early as the first month of life, and build a huge reservoir of love in their first year through compelling visual exchanges with everyone in their orbit. How do I know this? My mother taught me. One of her favorite reminiscences about my first year was of her daily excursion to a sunny Bronx street corner where a large encampment of baby carriages and mostly Jewish mothers gathered each day. Jewish mother love is the Grade A kind and flowed in abundance on that oasis of cement. My mother had named me after New York's beloved mayor, Jimmy Walker, and by unanimous vote of the encampment I was a future mayor. Not a bad way to start out in life.

The medical profession attracts three kinds of people: those who want to become rich, those who simply love science, and a clear majority who want to be helpful to their fellow man. A doctor's personal warmth and love for other humans is often what saves the day for patients in crisis. Hippocrates, himself, is my authority for this statement. In 640 BC, he wrote about the degree of personal goodness that doctors should try to achieve. He said they must live "Holy" lives as befits agents of the gods, and that sometimes this inner sanctity could, by itself, cure serious illness. Physicians have since tried to live up to this high standard of inner love for others by taking the Hippocratic Oath at graduation.

Medical education involves so much more than book learning. In the clinical years it calls upon teachers to show their students how to transmit important medical information in a heart to heart way. Watching how doctors talk with their patients in the clinics exposes students to the art of getting through with inner warmth. And it's not only how they talk, but also how they listen. Dr. Harold Jeghers, Professor of Medicine at Georgetown in the mid-fifties, introduced the idea of having his students at Tufts and Georgetown wear their names on their uniforms, along with the title Doctor, as they went about their work on the wards. He wanted them to learn at an early age how special doctors are in the minds of their patients. Sitting beside bed-ridden patients, and talking with them about their sickness, we discovered a unique kind of intimacy. Going home at night we found ourselves preoccupied with touching memories of the bedside conversations. It was the beginning of learning to carry patients around inside ourselves.

By taking an internship in internal medicine at Georgetown I had a chance to see some really great communicators in action. Dr. Jeghers was known affectionately as "Moose", because of his square jaw, rugged features, brevity of speech and strong integrity. He had been considered one of the high priests at "The Mecca"—the Harvard Group of Hospitals in Boston, along with those related to Boston University and Tufts. By recruiting all of his sub-specialists from "The Mecca", Georgetown

University Hospital had acquired the name of "The Harvard of the South". Dr. George Schreiner, a prime mover in development of the artificial kidney, came from the Peter Bent Brigham, as did Charles Hufnagel, surgical co-founder of cardiac valve operations. Larry Kyle in endocrinology, Charles Rath in hematology, and Irving Brick in gastro-enterology all came from hospitals in the Harvard group. His prize acquisition was Dr. W. Proctor Harvey, a former professor at Harvard and co-author of a leading textbook in cardiology. I made rounds with each of these men on a number of occasions. They were the leading practitioners in their specialties in Washington, and also nationally well known for published papers. Their individual personality styles were markedly different. Some were strongly opinionated, and aggressive, a couple even quick tempered. Others were soft-spoken and self-effacing. They were the same in one respect. When it came to meeting with patients their inner warmth was immediately in evidence and gave them easy access to details of illness. As they reviewed these with patients the latter became much better at self-observation, and were able to take in the explanations given them. It was possible for those of us who were observers to witness a strengthening of patients, a boost in self-confidence vis-a-vis their illness, and a commitment to treatment plans.

Proctor Harvey was easily the most admired and well-liked physician at Georgetown. When Dr. Jeghers had accepted my application for internship he told me that I was now relieved of any other obligations as a fourth year student, and was to spend my entire last four months as a Fellow with Dr. Harvey, seeing patients and going to conferences with him. It was the best four months of my professional life. Dr. Harvey's patients were many and varied, coming from every part of the country. All had serious heart disease, many were in danger of sudden death. Their encounters with Dr. Harvey's gentle manner, patient listening and sage advice displayed the healing power of inner warmth even in desperate life circumstances.

Dr. Harvey had only been at Georgetown for several months and two of his contributions had already improved clinical life around the hospital. Both speak of his passion for getting close to patients and even inside them. Auscultation, the art of listening to a human body with a stethoscope, was his forte. For years the trend in stethoscopes had been for longer and longer models, I suspect to allow for less bending on the part of physicians. Dr. Harvey introduced one with the shortest tubing any of us had ever seen, less than half the usual length. His use of it was a beautiful sight for it brought his head into close proximity with the patient's chest, and the caring look on his face revealed his intense absorption in the task of listening. His instrument soon acquired the facetious name of the Proctorscope, of course not implying any connection with the anal tool of similar name. It wasn't very long before all of the house staff had trimmed their stethoscopes down to Proctorscope size, a few exhibitionists even opting for four-inch tubing. Dr. Harvey was indeed the Sherlock Holmes of the chest, intent on not missing a single clue from the inside. Shortly after his arrival at Georgetown he took over a large janitorial closet on the medical floor to set up a listening post where doctors and nurses could go in their free time to hear his personal recordings of every type of cardiac pathology. A couple of easy chairs and a hi-fi speaker completed the gift of what he himself had heard from within the chests of several hundred patients. His listening post is still in operation, teaching young doctors and nurses the fine art and science of cardiac auscultation.

Dr. Charles Hufnagel was Dr. Harvey's counterpart in the surgical department and together they formed a perfect team for the diagnosis and repair of cardiac defects. Dr. Hufnagel had already acquired some fame for the first installation of a kidney transplant in an emergency operation at the Peter Bent Brigham. He had an assortment of artificial heart valves on hand for the first aortic valve replacement, and could also perform bypass surgery when necessary. Dr. Harvey shared in every final decision for surgery and had the leading role in managing post-operative crises. There were many of these tense moments in which the two professors met with their Fellows to map out a strategy for saving a life. The deep respect of these two men for one another was unmistakable and inspiring. Dr. Harvey's ability to have a calming effect on his partner, and on all of us, led some to think of him as the secret of Dr. Hufnagel's success.

About six months into internship, Dr. Harvey brought a patient with advanced chronic heart disease onto my ward at one in the morning. As he finished writing his orders, I told him that I had planned to stay on the ward through the night, and would be able to watch his patient closely and keep him informed. He thanked me, and said, "But I think I'll just sit up in the chair in his room. I'm afraid he may not make it and I want to be here for his family." They arrived at five am, just in time for final good-byes. Dr. Harvey had already taught me about as much cardiology as my mind could manage, but he gave me a lesson in caring that night that I will never forget.

Working with doctors who have that kind of dedication has given me a love of internal medicine and respect for internists that has remained strong until this day. Every Friday morning at seven-thirty, Sibley Memorial Hospital, a satellite of Georgetown, hosts a one-hour conference on the latest topics and new developments in internal medicine. I rarely miss it. A few of my old supervisors from internship days are still in attendance, along with a number of men and women from all the specialties who are regulars. It's a sure tonic, a perfect way to round out a week of practice on a positive note. I feel quite strongly that psychiatrists should keep up with the latest medical information on every kind of problem. It's amazing how often one of my patients will make an offhand comment that registers with something I've heard in Friday's meeting and leads me to suggest they talk it over with their family doctor.

After internship, I spent two years of training in psychiatry and neurology at Georgetown, and then I heard the call of "The Mecca", the single most important event in my development as a psychiatrist. Georgetown's residency in psychiatry was only a few years old, but it had a consultant who was one of the most highly regarded psychiatrists in this country, Dr. Leo Bartemeyer. Dr. Bartemeyer was President of the American Psychoanalytic Association and even had the credential of having worked as a general practitioner in his preparation for this position. He caught me by surprise one day with the observation that having spent three years at Georgetown I would do well to get some training elsewhere. He suggested that I get into one of the many programs in Boston. I asked him which one he thought was best and he said, "Well the Beth Israel, of course, but that one's really hard to get into. It's affiliated with Harvard, and they only take one or two new people a year out of about forty applicants." He went on to say, "You know they call that place the Camelot of American Psychiatry because of the high morale of its staff. If you want to apply there, I'll write a letter of recommendation to Grete Bibring, the Chief psychiatrist. It's a long shot, but worth it. I do think you'd have a much better chance to get into the programs of Boston University or Tufts."

Dr. Bibring interviewed every one of the applicants herself, and I must have been the last one because of my late application. A few days later, I had a phone call from her telling me of my acceptance. At the time, I thought it must have come about because of Dr. Bartemeyer's letter, and also because of my Irish background in a city with so many more of the same ancestry. A few years afterward I was told by one of

Dr. Bibring's top assistants that that wasn't the case at all. "She makes every selection by herself", he said, "on the basis of her interview. She has only two criteria for her final choices: Does she like the person and would they fit in." We must have had more resonance of our inner warmth than I had realized.

3

The Camelot of American Psychiatry Boston's Beth Israel Hospital

When I look back on those two years at Camelot there's only one word that comes to mind: extraordinary. They were just extraordinary. It was like a whole new world had opened up before me, and each day afforded a fresh opportunity for intimate encounters with other people. For one thing, the staff had no secrets from one another. Almost everyone had been in psychoanalysis and they shared their innermost thoughts quite freely. Petty rivalries were non-existent, and if you were having some trouble with a tough case you had many colleagues with a ready ear and good advice.

Beth Israel's psychiatric department had another pseudonym beside Camelot. It was also called "Freudland on the Brookline", after Brookline Avenue and the department's distinctive lineage. Two of Freud's own trainees, Drs. Grete and Edward Bibring, had rescued psychoanalysis from its ivory tower and put it to work at Beth Israel as a tool for easing the tensions of every day living. Their outreach went in many directions—to children, parents, teachers, lawyers and clergy, but over and above all to doctors and their patients. Using their understanding of the role of the emotions in medical illness they had created a consultation service with a ninety-five percent success rate in changing the behavior patterns of "uncooperative" medical and surgical patients. Getting through with inner warmth was a way of life at Beth Israel. Every resident in psychiatry was also involved in providing long-term support for patients with serious organic illness. The "B.I." had the most well respected psychiatric service of any general hospital in the country.

Dr. Grete Bibring taught her resident physicians that the first requirement in their field was to be a good and caring doctor. She understood that it was quite normal for people to have fears about psychiatry, especially psychoanalytic psychiatry with its ominous reputation for exposing the demons in each of us. At Beth Israel she made it clear that the main function of her department was to enhance medical and surgical care in every area of the hospital. Her instructions to her residents were simple: "Whenever you have some free time, go up to the ward where you are assigned and get to know the doctors, nurses and patients better. Let them see that that's where you do your work. When you learn how to talk with them in their language, they'll want you on their team."

Psychiatric consultation became a new kind of experience for all concerned. Typically, psychiatrists were introduced to patients as "a doctor on the hospital staff who is interested in how your treatment is going." A friendly handshake, an opening comment like, "Well now, how have you been doing here?" would invite the patients' candid appraisal of their progress or lack of it, and their anger about staff ineptitude. They would speak of the frustration and pain of their illness, and of their fears, including especially the fear of death. Often they recounted how they had handled past crises, both medical and otherwise. Most of these consultations were conducted without apparent awareness on the patients' part that they were talking with a psychiatrist. If asked about our specialty, the answer would be, "I'm a psychiatrist, but with a special interest in medical problems and how normal people manage them."

Dr. Bibring trained her staff to listen carefully to what they were being told, to remember the patient's exact words, phrasing and sequences of topics, to be supportive and empathic at all times, and to intrude as little as possible into the free flow of the patient's communication. An old medical rule of thumb said that fifteen percent of all medical treatments were doomed to failure because of the patient's lack of cooperation with their physician's prescribed regimen. Both nurses and doctors at Beth Israel were very sensitive to this danger, and quick to call for psychiatric consultation even when the evidence for lack of cooperation was subtle. The success rate of Dr. Bibring's consultation service for these sometimes life-threatening situations was a well known and often discussed fact around the hospital.

Frequently a chance remark would reveal the secret of a patient's personality structure. Dr. Bibring's whole approach was based on finding that secret, the answer to the question "How does this person get along?" Most people are dominated by one of three kinds of anxiety: separation or abandonment anxiety, fear of loss of approval, or bodily damage anxiety. As an example, I remember a fireman who came in with a major heart attack and was told by the doctors and nurses that he had to remain completely in bed for two weeks (the standard treatment in those days). He absolutely refused to do this and came walking down to the nursing station every few minutes to show that he was all right. His opening comment to me was "I carried a guy out of a building just last week who was over 250 pounds. Now they're trying to tell me I have to stay in bed."

I said, "You know the hardest thing I can think of for an active man like yourself is to ask if he can stay still, and remain in bed for two weeks. But that's what I'm going to ask you to try to do. It won't be easy, but I think you can do it, and that way you'll be able to go back to work much sooner. Now you're going to be getting intravenous medications for the next several days and I want you to be in charge of your own IV so the nurses won't have to keep running in to check on it. They'll tell you about how many drops a minute are good and you can keep adjusting it until it runs out." We shook hands and his firm grip and eye to eye contact told me we had an agreement. His emphasis on his bodily strength had made it easy to identify his anxiety—fear of bodily damage. He loved challenges and had to be helped to see that staying in bed for two weeks was the biggest challenge in his life. The unspoken message he had heard was that these doctors really understand what kind of a guy I am.

Supposing he had said "I'm afraid of dying. I need to be around other people." We might then have surmised that his trips to the nursing station were based on separation anxiety. He would have been told, "Don't worry about the IVs, the nurses will be in to check on you regularly and they'll look after your IV. If you need them for anything you can use the call button. And, while you're asleep tonight they'll be coming in often just to keep watch, and they won't awaken you." Cardiac patients with fear of loss of approval anxiety were told they could put their two weeks in bed to good use by making up lists of things needed by each member of their family so they could be ready to get going on these when they got home.

I remember thinking at the time that this was the most sophisticated and effective psychological approach to a normal and practical human problem that I had ever seen. It was that, but I now recognize it was much more. After all, it means a great deal to someone who is frightened and angry, and maybe fed-up and furious enough to attack any and all doctors, to find a physician who can accept his or her rage, and not strike back or run away, who is ready to listen and try to understand. There comes a moment when the modern specialist must behave in the very human way of the old family doctor. Once good person to person contact is reestablished, the patient's rage gives way to relief. It is then that the physician ceases to seem the persecutor, and becomes instead an ally and friend.

Very often the consultation would lead to an on-going relationship between doctor and patient. My first consultation was with a teenager who had a defective clotting mechanism and recurrent bleeding episodes. He was well known on the medical wards because his frequent fistfights led to an average of six to eight hospitalizations each year for episodes of internal bleeding. His fame was also based on his antisocial behavior in the hospital, which had earned him the nickname of "Tommy, the Terrible". Tommy hated nurses. He leered, glowered and cursed at them. He whispered caustic comments, barely audible, about their height, weight, breasts, legs, and buttockses. He also fired occasional spitballs at them. In our first meeting he opened with the comment: "You look too young to be a doctor here. Most of my doctors are stupid old men." I asked how he got into so many fights, and he told me about his membership in a gang with pride in their exploits, and little apparent regret for his injuries. I told him I had a friend who was a well-known gang leader in the Bronx. He had been hired by a swimming pool where I worked as a lifeguard, to walk around the pool in a lifeguard uniform even though he couldn't swim a stroke. He was enormously successful at preserving the peace there. We traded some stories about gang wars, and I told him I'd be back in the morning with more time to talk. The next day he told me he really enjoyed "rapping with" me, and said it was the first time he had ever "rapped with" a doctor. He said he had some questions about a bone marrow procedure the doctors wanted to perform. We talked about these and he gave his "o.k." Over time we were able to talk about many of the questions he had had about his illness and treatment, and there was a noticeable improvement in his behavior on the ward. Later he came by the psychiatry department any time he had an out-patient medical appointment over the next two years, and always asked for "Doc". Our ad hoc rap sessions touched on many personal matters besides medical problems. During this time he had only two minor bleeding episodes, gave up fighting and returned to school. Our collaborative efforts had brought his bleeding tendency under pretty good control for the first time in his life.

Another patient, Jeannie, a fifty year-old married woman, had a rare neurological disease whose rapid downhill course had wrecked her relationships with her doctors and her husband. She was pleased to have a doctor assigned to her who was "here to listen and was not going to try to force me to take any more medicines that don't work." She said that she was tired of fighting with doctors, and only wanted "to get back on the same wavelength like it used to be" with her husband. I found our meetings to be very enjoyable. She had a wonderful sense of humor that she brought to bear on her illness, and hospital life, and she undertook to enlarge my Jewish vocabulary, teaching me the subtle nuances of many new words and phrases. My favorite one was "uberschrein" that referred to a tactic she often used. She said "that was when you're having an argument with someone and you know you are wrong so you shout louder than them and don't give them a chance to talk." She was having problems in her sexual relationship with her husband that had been brought on by her illness, and she found these easier to talk about with her doctor than with her spouse. With encouragement, she finally became able to take them up with him, and the discussion led to a return of warmth in their relationship.

The most disturbing symptom of Jeannie's disease had been the development of a "flapping tremor", a coarse type of flailing movement of the arms that had made it impossible to write letters or even sign her name. After awhile she noticed that our weekly meetings were "having a calming effect" on her anger towards doctors, and soon thereafter on her flapping tremor. It stopped completely. She became able to write letters to her family and friends and sign her name on any necessary occasion. The exchanges of warmth with a doctor had quieted her anger and at least slowed the relentless progress of her illness. About two months after my departure from Beth Israel I received a letter from her in perfect penmanship thanking me for the cure of her flapping tremor and telling me it was no longer necessary to uberschein.

I was fascinated by this phase of our work at Beth Israel. There were no carefully formulated interpretations—and no deep insights—just a plain old friendly relationship with a doctor who was an auxiliary to the medical team. Over a two-year period I saw a number of patients who had clear improvements in their organic illness from our joint efforts. I asked myself could it really be that a serious physical illness could be kept at bay for a much longer time by the simple sharing of inner warmth with a doctor. I was determined to work on this question further when I got out into my own private practice. Two of my classmates who were internists helped me get started on this pursuit almost immediately upon my return to Washington.

Dr. Jack Maher, a nephrologist and protegee of Dr. George Schreiner, asked me to see a patient with a severe lupus that had damaged his kidneys and was progressive. He was apologetic about the referral, saying, "I don't think this man is your usual kind of patient. He doesn't have any kind of psychiatric problem yet, but he's entering the terminal phase and I have to break the news to him. His college classmates had a yearbook poll with lots of categories and they named him as the "most dependent person." I think he's going to need some extra support over the next few months but you won't have to see him long. He's only got about three or four months to live."

The patient, a likeable man named Hank, began a period of once a week psychotherapy with me immediately. His college classmates had been quite right about his personality structure, but fortunately his physician had been wrong about his prognosis. Hank was still alive twenty-five years later, when he was able to overcome his dependency on me, and move to a retirement community in another part of the country. Did his psychotherapy prolong his life? Dr. Maher, who was a well known expert on lupus, was certain that it had. With an hour each week to talk about all the minute details of his illness and how it affected his life it was possible to get into the disease process itself with him. It was a case of delivering an extra supply of loving energies to where they were needed the most, right into the area producing an overflow of frustration and anger. Feelings like that are a natural conse-quence of a life-threatening illness, but their presence aggravates the physical damage of the disease itself.

Dr. Jim Nugent referred the second patient, Doctor E. or Mrs E. as she preferred to be called. She was a brilliant scientist, and loving mother, who initiated psychotherapy after she was told that she had a chronic form of leukemia with a prognosis of death in five years. She had had a successful psychoanalysis with another psychiatrist many years before, and reasoned that psychotherapy might prolong her life. She, too, had a twenty-five year period of therapy, and led a very pro-ductive life before finally succumbing to her illness at the age of sev-enty-seven. She was the ideal patient of every psychiatrist's dreams.

Mrs. E was a devotee of Freud, but much more than that she loved her life, loved her husband and children, loved her creative hobbies, and loved her scientific career. She talked freely about her old neurotic problems, and was very perceptive when they intruded into any of the important areas of her life. If her creativity was temporarily stalled she studied that. When she became angry with her husband, children or colleagues she worked on that. But more than anything else she kept a constant vigil on her illness. Alert to the least sign of it worsening, she drew on her scientific mind and carefully researched the latest information about its treatment.

She arranged a number of consultations with physicians other than her internist, but always subjected these to review in our meetings lest her anger and frustration with her own doctor interfere with making the right moves about her treatment. In this way she was able to preserve the good relationship she had with her internist who attended her until her death. Mrs. E's sharing of warmth in our work together helped to keep all her loving relationships intact, including that with her internist, and allowed her to neutralize the anger component of her illness. I am sure this was a factor in her lengthy survival. The answer to my question from Beth Israel days about the long-term value of shared inner warmth for improving the outlook of serious illness turned out to be a res ipsa loquitur.

The concept of alternative medicine was not yet a popular item back then, but Grete Bibring had found a way to harness the inner warmth of her staff into a therapeutic dynamo that came at organic illness from a different direction than drugs. For many it was more powerful than drugs and gave them a dominance over their illness. It drew on the most elemental force in human nature, the limitless resource of shared inner warmth. Here was the precursor and often the basic ingredient of alternative medicine. In retrospect, Dr. Grete Bibring deserved the recognition of a Nobel Prize in medicine for her highly successful consultation service.

The rich tradition of Boston as a medical center where the training of young doctors was a high priority, and conferences everywhere were open to everyone, was deeply in-grained in Dr. Bibring's Fellows. Our service was the principal resource for the Harvard University School of Medicine both for the treatment of its faculty, and the instruction of its medical students. Fellows spent a great deal of time sharing clinical experiences with students and also with one another. Case conferences were held two or three nights each week in the homes of our supervisors. These were wonderfully warm occasions, with an open bar, desserts and in the case of Dr. Marty Berezin some family chamber music to begin the evening.

Child psychiatry was in its infancy then with only a few approved training centers around the country. Boston was the only city with more than one of these, and it had five including Beth Israel's program, under the direction of Dr. Henry Wermer. In my second year of fellowship I opted to spend more time in the child division and Henry became my mentor. It was a good move. With his ebullient Viennese personality and clinical brilliance he brought joy into the lives of children, parents and colleagues. He orchestrated the union of the five training centers into the Harvard Consortium for Child Psychiatry, with the finest faculty in the world. His own program maintained a close liaison with Anna Freud's clinic in London, giving all of us a chance to spend a few days there, making rounds with her and attending her case conferences.

The "Dean" of Boston's child psychoanalysts was Dr. Lydia Dawes, and she was also my favorite supervisor out in the community. She was a close friend of Anna Freud, and Dr. Eric Erickson, and shared many anecdotes about their work with children. One of the cases I presented to her was Danny, a six year old youngster, who tended to be quite rough on his younger siblings. He was so open and verbal that I always had a lot of material to review with her. In several of his treatment sessions I noticed "sudden thoughts" about the hidden meanings of his play behavior, and was tempted to comment on these to him. I reported them to Dr. Dawes, and said that I had hesitated to make the comments to him because I thought it too early in his treatment. A few weeks later, after another similar episode, she said "Now let's talk about your sudden thoughts." To my surprise she reviewed them all in great detail, and then she said, "You know, your sudden thoughts were all the product of your intuition, and I believe they were all exactly correct. You have a wonderful intuition, and that's a great gift. From now on, whenever you have a sudden thought you should share it, and not just with Danny, but with any patient." I have since had many occasions to take her advice, always to the benefit of my patients, and with fond memories of her whenever I do.

Danny loved to draw when we were in the playroom and over a year's time he produced a remarkable series of pictures that charted his progress in treatment. They began with totally dark, nocturnal skies that were filled with soldiers in airplanes, parachutes, and on the ground, all firing bullets at one another. Then he started to introduce a little sunlight to the top of the scene, with a sun that became an increasingly prominent part of the picture. The darkness gave way to sunshine and beautiful blue skies, with a smiling mother, father and three sons walking along, holding hands and headed to a church. In the real world, he became very fond of his two brothers and proud to assume the role of a big brother protector.

The leading psychoanalysts of Boston each provided many hours a week to various aspects of the program and worked pro bono for the opportunity to teach and to learn. Clinical conferences were held in abundance, often attended by Dr. Bibring. When she was present she would speak last, after many brilliant and insightful comments by her colleagues. This was the moment that all in attendance were waiting for. In her soft and gentle voice she had a way of introducing us to what was usually a totally new perspective, intensely warm and human, into the emotional life of the patient under discussion. She would enlarge on many of the excellent comments already made, and weave them into a pattern that showed new connections between what had been said by others. She could disagree with someone's thinking, but always in a way that protected that person's ego, giving due credit to the reasons for their speculation, but reshaping it with additional observations of her own. There was an awesome quality to her final assessment of a patient, richly enhanced by the warmth and respect she had for a human being she had not even met. Most of us regarded her as the greatest psychiatrist in the world, and considered her husband the most important psychoanalytic theorist since Freud.

It was our special privilege as Fellows to have regular, forty-five minute, supervisory sessions with Dr. Bibring. In an intimate moment near the end of a session, Dr. Bibring asked me the kind of question that only she could ask. To a lay person it might seem like one of the most obvious questions in the world. And yet, I had never heard it asked by one psychiatrist of another, nor had I heard one of my colleagues volunteer the answer on his own. She said, "Dr. Ryan, who is your favorite kind of patient?"

It may be that I had some idea that psychiatrists weren't supposed to have favorite patients, or that we just didn't talk about things like that. Perhaps I felt having favorite patients would cloud our cherished objectivity or neutrality. In any case I regarded her question as very important to me, and I wanted to be sure I gave the most candid self-assessment possible. I asked her if I might take a moment to think, and during the next minute or two I ran through the rolodex of all my categories of patients, thinking of various persons in each and watching my own feeling response carefully.

She had given me permission to have favorite patients, and I enjoyed the task she had set forth. Hysterics, people with a prominent sexual influence in their make-up, came to mind first. They were the most talked about, and many would admit, the most fun to work with. Compulsives were less emotional, more orderly and cerebral. Treating them was a challenging and worthwhile task but not a favorite one. Dependent persons were sometimes draining but often warm and quite lovable. Borderlines were a difficult new category that had won my enthusiasm because of supervision by Dr. Arnold Modell, one of the pioneers in the field. And, finally, children where we once again had world class supervisors like Drs. Lydia Dawes and Henry Wermer, and where the results of therapy were often spectacular.

It seemed to me I had lots of favorite patients but no clear-cut front-runner as to type, when suddenly three figures emerged from a shadowy corner of my mind. They were schizophrenics, two women and a young man. When I had met them in my first year of residency at D.C.General, they looked like certain candidates for St. Elizabeth's. They had escaped this unhappy fate for a variety of administrative reasons and been assigned to me for long-term care. At the outset all three appeared to be hopelessly withdrawn from the real world, and yet, slowly, slowly, by almost invisible increments, they had begun to inch their way back. During the week before I won my own freedom from D. C. General, they were discharged from that institution and embarked on what proved to be a year of out-patient psychotherapy at the Georgetown University Hospital. There were no moments of spectacular insights, but these three patients never missed appointments, and they worked hard at the tasks of finding jobs, creating a small social life, and getting along with their families. When I received the good news of my acceptance at Beth Israel, the patients and I began a six-month period of saying goodbye and getting them ready to continue with a new therapist at Georgetown.

One of the two women was just twenty and had lived at home in seclusion with disparaging "voices" that told her not to go outside for any reason. She was able to find a job and managed some dates with men, although she had the delusion that I had arranged both the job and dates for her. We had to carefully undo the grip of this delusion so that she could proceed in forging a life of her own and accepting her transfer to another doctor.

The second woman had already endured thirteen hospitalizations in the preceding fifteen years and teetered constantly on the brink of her fourteenth. Her life was a series of recurrent crises that taxed the rescue capacities of the social service department and at times exhausted her therapist. She managed to stay out of the hospital by the slender reed of her newfound capacity to question her paranoid delusions. At the time of my departure she was in her sixth "newest job".

The young man had succumbed to a classical dementia praecox in his last year of high school. This was the old name for schizophrenia when it was believed to come on most often in adolescence. His illness had begun with a tormented period of compulsive masturbation. Soon angry male and female "voices" were threatening him with punishment for his "sinful life." As he emerged from his social withdrawal during out-patient treatment, he became a daily churchgoer and eventually joined a religious order.

The answer to Dr. Bibring's question came with trepidation and surprise. Even as the words "I think I like schizophrenics the best" were being said, I was asking myself "Why?" Of greater concern was how she might react to my choice, since none of my patients at Beth Israel had been schizophrenic.

Her response was swift, sure and full of warmth. "Oh I'm glad. You would be very good with schizophrenics. And you know, we need to learn so much more about this illness. It is such a hardship for the patients and their families. Freud always thought that psychoanalysis would one day solve the riddle of schizophrenia. His greatest disappointment was that he couldn't do this himself. He was sure that the solution of the mystery of schizophrenia would provide a wealth of new information about human nature.

For the next few weeks I wondered a good bit about the implications of my comment to Dr. Bibring. I had already decided to return to Washington and enter private practice. Above all else I wanted to be a teacher like my mentors at Beth Israel. A part-time job on the faculty at Georgetown seemed to be the best way to reach this goal, and a request for a place at the University Hospital had already been submitted. To my profound disappointment none was available. I was, however, offered a teaching and administrative position at D.C.General. Unsure whether or not to accept, I discussed the matter with Dr. Bibring. "Well," she said, "The most important thing about any job is whether it will allow you enough time to have your own analysis and to pursue your psychoanalytic studies. It sounds like this position would be excellent in that regard. Beyond that, you want to be in a place where you could put your analytic knowledge to good use, and I think a hospital for acute schizophrenics would be just such a place. It would be a challenge, but that's how we learn new things. You know that you like to work with schizophrenic patients. Don't be afraid to follow your heart. And remember Freud's promise, that the understanding of schizophrenia would cast a new light on human nature."

My Oracle at Delphi had spoken in a clear and unambiguous way. I was ready to leave Camelot with something much more important than new knowledge and skills. It was with a sense of purpose, a dual mission: to learn more about the healing power of inner warmth, and to solve the mystery of schizophrenia. Grete Bibring, herself, had given me this assignment. It was a lifetime task that has culminated in this book.

4

New man on the staff of D.C. General

I was still miffed at Georgetown's Department of Psychiatry for farming me out to D.C.General, as I drove there on that hot summer morning. I had had such wonderful daydreams about starting a consultation service in the University Hospital, and now I was going to a place where almost no one got better. It was time for a reality check on my hopes to find an explanation for schizophrenia. There would be no shortage of clinical material for the endeavor. D.C.General took in over three thousand patients a year, and sixty percent of these were suffering from acute schizophrenia. The problem in studying their illnesses would be the rapid turnover. From my days as a first year resident there I knew that we operated as a revolving door to St. Elizabeth's, the "state hospital" for Washington, D.C. Patients could only remain with us for one day to two weeks before their legal commitment to St. E's.

On the other hand, D.C.G.H. had a notable asset, the seasoned and dedicated nursing staff. Helen Shea, Chief Nurse, was a kind and wise administrator who had the total respect of everyone in the building. Chris Welch and Rosie Gibson were Charge Nurses having great rapport with patients, doctors and nursing assistants alike. Chris weighed a few pounds less than a hundred, yet had little fear of violent patients whom she could usually subdue with sweetness. Rosie had the same kind of inner warmth and evident concern for the well being of others.

Leroy Alston and David Jerry had been nursing assistants there for fifteen years and were the first line of defense against violent patients, reining them in with admirable courage and skill. The staff had lived through many years of little hope for patient recoveries, and now they had the dawn of hope with the new tranquilizing drug, Thorazine. It could put violent patients to sleep instantly. It was from my memories of the heroic efforts of this whole group that I drew my own hope as we started our days together once again.

The Chief Psychiatrist was Dr. John Schultz, a capable clinician and superb bureaucrat. He had been on the job for four years and in that time had pushed plans for a brand new hospital through the Medical Society, the University Medical Schools, the Army Corps of Engineers and a host of local politicians and advocacy groups. The grand opening had taken place just four weeks before my arrival. John had given me a fancy title, Chief of Forensic Psychiatry, meaning I would appear in court for patients who had criminal charges against them. Along with it came an office with a beautiful view of the Anacostia River, and an anteroom for my secretary, Mrs. Audrey Buckner. She was considered by many to be the best secretary in the hospital. During those first years at D.C.General I spent a lot of time testifying in court under the new "Durham Rule" for the insanity defense. Since this rule required a psychiatrist to study the past mental condition of a person, at the time of their crime, the length of evaluations had gone up from two hours to twenty or more. The longer assessment time had allowed us to find a number of people who had been overtly schizophrenic at the time of their crime, and had recovered subsequently while in jail. We were forced to the painful conclusion that the jail had a much better recovery rate than our own state of the art hospital.

What was the D.C.General Psychiatric Pavilion like in the early sixties? We were a 240-bed hospital taking in anyone who had had an acute mental breakdown in the Greater Washington area. They came in right off the streets, sometimes in police vans or ambulances, or surrounded by several family members. Often four or five policemen would be engaged in a struggle with a patient right on our doorstep. One or two patients were in locked security rooms where they had only a mattress, and urinated on the floors. There were usually three or four tied down in beds with leather restraints on all four extremities. They shouted curses that shook the walls and ceilings, and rattled their beds with violent muscular contractions until we could give them a large injection of Thorazine to put them to sleep. When the wards were quiet, thanks to Thorazine, there was an eerie coldness that permeated the building due to the deep withdrawal of our patients from other people and the world. Their inner warmth was at ebb tide with none to share with their fellow humans. Patients were lodged on all-male or all-female wards while awaiting their likely transfer to St. Elizabeth's seven thousand—bed hospital. All of them wore only pajamas, a measure believed to quiet them down, and make an effort to escape unlikely. Many wandered the halls aimlessly, like robots, muttering delusional thoughts or trying to converse with "hidden voices" that were tormenting them. The biggest problem was the danger of unpredictable outbursts of violence against one another, or staff members.

D.C.General had created a shiny new hospital, but I felt uncomfortable in it. It had too many features that made one feel like being in a prison. The heavy metal security screens were more than escape proof. They were overwhelming. The elevators were locked, the nursing stations locked and walled in by thick glass, and every ward was secured by a locked door along with a number of locked bedrooms.

5

Discovery of the warming point

My most important teaching assignment was to conduct twice-weekly new admission ward rounds with eight medical students, and one or two resident doctors. They were free to pick the patients to be seen, and always selected those whom they had already found difficult or impossible to interview. Thus we could expect to encounter some that were mute as well as some who were volcanically verbal, some who were coldly hostile and others seething with rage. Many would present with only the classic flat affect and mental chaos of schizophrenia.

For the first couple of years at this task I followed each interview with a brief talk to the students and residents summarizing the wide range of symptoms and signs we had just seen. Then we'd move rapidly on to the next encounter. Sometime during the fourth year of rounding I began to notice a strange new feeling arising within myself and taking over my whole being. I felt determined to pierce the dense fog of psychosis, and find some spark of rationality. Where this profound urge was coming from I didn't know at the time, but we'll get to the answer in two chapters.

One morning our rounds group descended on one of the male units to find an urgent problem awaiting us. The two resident physicians were waiting for us at the front door and ushered us into an alcove for some private conversation. "I'm afraid we've got a tiger by the tail," said one. "We've got a man who came in yesterday as a voluntary patient from the main admitting office without any background information on his chart. We don't know what he told them over there. Yesterday he began talking in a word salad all day long and then this morning he began to say a few sentences. They all have to do with going out. He said he wants to leave and that there is no problem. He won't really say why he came in. I don't think we should let him go, but then we would have to file some commitment papers, and what do we tell the Mental Health Commission? Right now all we could say is he just looks dangerous and that isn't enough."

"Besides", said the other resident, "This fellow looks kind of mean, just the type who would sue us if we tried to keep him here."

And so we met with the patient, eight white-coated figures that crowded into a small office with a grim and ashen faced patient. He began by saying that he wanted to leave right now—although the tone of his voice conveyed none of the urgency of the words "right now". He spoke in the depersonalized monotone of schizophrenia and it almost seemed as though his words were barely escaping through his tight lips. His taut jaw was secured by his masseter muscles, which rippled in a constant state of commotion.

"I know about psychiatry", the patient volunteered. "I took a course in psychology once. There is the ego, the superego and the lid."

To which I responded: "You know, what you say is not quite right. The ego and superego ARE the lid, and I think that that is what you're having trouble with right now. You're afraid you might not be able to keep the lid on."

The patient broke out in laughter, at first a bit hollow, but changing quickly into a warm chuckle. He smiled, and then provided us with a brief and earnest account of his lifelong struggle with voices that mocked him and threatened him with bodily harm. He had purchased a rifle for self-protection, but recently had begun to notice other voices that were suggesting that he use the weapon on some of his neighbors. And so he had taken refuge with us chiefly to guard against his own murderous impulses, but now he was finding that various other patients aroused his rage, especially his roommates, whom he had urges to kill. Within a few minutes he and I were able to agree on a treatment plan. He would take certain medications. If he had a rage storm, he could talk with staff members or spend time alone in an unlocked room. His wife would be free to visit as he saw fit.

Following the ancient medical tradition, our rounds group huddled briefly before seeing the next patient, to discuss what we had just observed. There was a rather immediate consensus that there had been a turning point in the interview with this last patient, at which a dramatic change occurred. It had happened during the patient's laughter. This was clear from his whole manner and speech from that point on. The gist of the students' comments was that the patient had been cold and strange, distant and aloof, or off in his own world at the outset, then warmed considerably at what proved to be a turning point. He subsequently became quite reasonable and cooperative, or almost normal except for some funny ideas. One of them noted that he even seemed to be questioning some of his own delusions, and another said "You really got to him when you made that remark about keeping the lid on, maybe it was because you used his own word."

What is it that makes a teacher suddenly pause and take some time to review his own efforts? I am sure the good ones do this quite often, but I must confess it had not been a regular part of my own routine until this very meeting. Whatever the reason, the mental tape of our session continued to play on, and it began to resonate with the memories of other post-interview discussions.

In recent weeks the rounds group had begun to speak of a "warming point" quite frequently. By this they were referring to when a schizophrenic suddenly warms up, and becomes more accessible and cooperative. I was starting to have some success in convincing patients of their need to remain in the hospital. A comment such as "You sound like you're confused" would draw the reply of "Yes, I am". I could use this exchange to gain an accord about staying. These glimmers of rational thinking were not as striking as the one just seen. The words "A warming point, then rational thinking" became lodged in my mind like a glowing ember that would not burn out.

The students had become the teachers. "They're trying to tell you something", I reasoned, "and you have to listen to them. They're trying to tell you that this is the most important thing that happens when you get together with these patients, and you've got to think about it some more and explain what it means."

The warming point in schizophrenia was clearly a very magical moment. It was like a key that opened a door to a rational part of a patient's mind. If there was one thing I had learned in my brief legal career it was how different two witnesses could be in their perception of the same event. Lawyers made fortunes on this truism. But here was an experience that eight or ten young clinicians were describing in exactly the same language, especially as to the timing of the occurrence. I could look backward four years or even one to an era when there would have been eight differing versions of the same scene, each one with its own catalogue of bizarre elements. Now they were in lockstep about a sign of life and rationality just observed.

The warming point was very much a two way happening and that had to be the reason for our unanimity of perception. In the warming point I was getting through to the patient and he or she was getting through to each one of us. We were obviously going through a great human linking experience although I wasn't very much impressed with that aspect at the time. My mind was on what it might mean for the hospital.

It was exciting to think about. Could it really be that we had identified a therapeutic transaction that would work for more of our patients? How many more? Might we some day close the revolving door to St. Elizabeth's? That seemed unlikely with only 240 beds and over 3000 admissions a year, but who knows? For now, the most important question was how do we get to the warming point?

I shared these thoughts with the rounds group in our next meeting, hoping for some answers on the latter point. "Well", Dr. Ryan, said one of the med students, "It seems to me you keep trying a lot of leads. If one doesn't work then you go to another. You seem to be looking for something the patient might be even a tiny bit interested in, but then you never know what that's going to be. It could be a lot of different things. You don't give up easily. Maybe that's what is most important."

"With some patients it seems like maybe you wear down their resistance", said another, "until you finally get a topic that both of you can talk about. It may be a very short conversation but that's when they warm up. You need to find some more patients like the lid man. You got through to him bigtime." He was absolutely right. One good case was not enough. We still had a lot to learn.

The "lid man", as he now became known to the students and residents alike, made a rapid recovery in the next three weeks. He asked to be in a room by himself for about an hour on each of the first two days, and came out on his own reporting that he felt better. He liked to make jokes about getting the lid back on, but took the purchase of his rifle and urges to use it quite seriously. He was shocked to think that his long-term fears of people could have erupted into the urge to kill, and he instructed his wife to give the rifle to the National Guard.

He had been unemployed and living off a pension for several months, but decided, with his doctor's help, that idleness had been one of his problems. Accordingly, after discharge, he got a job as a sacristan in a church, and was very pleased with his new occupation. He continued to see the resident physician at weekly intervals for the next few months and then in brief monthly meetings to discuss medication.

His hospitalization had lasted a little under three weeks and during this time the search for more lid men was underway in earnest. Just before his departure I happened to stop by a female ward one morning at seven and found two of our best residents, Joe Sebastian and Walt Anderson, having coffee. "We've got a good patient for your rounds group today", Joe said, "but you'll have to get your gang up here in a hurry. We'll be shipping her over to St. E's on a direct transfer later in the morning. "She's a tough one", he added, with Walt nodding in agreement. "She's elusive and evasive, looks paranoid, and I'm sure is hearing voices, but we can't get a thing out of her. She works for the XYZ Drugstore chain."

"Oh" said I, "and how do you know that/"

"Well she sure didn't tell me," he replied. "She must have mentioned it to one of the nurses".

"Let's go see her now," I said. "I'd like to speak with her about her job."

The patient was already in the hallway as we approached her, a slender pajama clad woman in her late forties. Her facial expression, which had been blank from a distance, grew etched with fear as we drew near. I introduced myself—told her that we wanted to talk with her a little bit—and said that I had been told by her doctor that she worked for the XYZ Drugstore chain.

Without a trace of feeling in her voice, she began to mumble that she worked in the Jay Street store at the lunch counter. She then added in almost the same tone, that she had worked for the chain for seventeen years, and during that time had been assigned to only two places. She identified the second of these by its street name and said that she had been there for the first eight years. I sensed a note of pride in her intonation of the word seventeen, although it was a barely detectable nuance of feeling.

"I've been to both of those stores", I told her with enthusiasm, "although never at the lunch hour. I used to buy my garden supplies in that first place you worked in. They really have a big garden section in the back".

"Yes, they do," she said with a slight accent on the "do". "I go back there sometimes to buy plants."

It was my turn now and I began to sense the beginning of a roll. "You have a larger paperback collection where you work now, don't you?

"Yes, that's for the girls who go to Trinity College, and the mothers who drive their kids to school. They like to come in for coffee and talk about the kids. Then they do the book section. The college girls don't sit down at the counter. They just stand around and talk. Then they buy some cosmetics before they look at the books.

It was clear she liked her fleeting contacts with these people. They occurred in a predictable and reliable fashion and were a steady source of pleasure. She also liked the very physical structure of her store, which we discussed in some detail, aisle by aisle. After several minutes, I said, "Your work is very important for you, isn't it?"

"It sure is. It's my life", she replied, with genuine conviction.

"You know", I said, "It sounds like we ought to be trying to help you get back there as soon as possible". She met my gaze, nodded and said an emphatic "Yes". Her flatness of affect was gone. "What brought you to this hospital?" was my final question.

Without losing the spark generated by our discussion of her job, she began to share with me the details of her illness. "Some strange things have been happening in my neighborhood for the past six or seven weeks," she said. "People have been talking about me and looking at me funny. I've been hearing messages over the television about me, mostly at night. I get real nervous. I mean just plain scared." She drew a deep breath and continued. "Someone in the apartment building has a big machine that plays right into my room—right across the walls. It's saying I'm a homosexual, only I'm not, and I hear voices saying the same thing and other nasty rumors all the time. But at night it's the worst, and I can't sleep right any more."

"Did something else go wrong in your life several weeks ago?" I asked.

"No", she said slowly, "only me and my boyfriend broke up, but I don't want to talk about that right now."

"A break-up can be very painful and upsetting," I said.

"Yes", she murmured.

"You may not feel like it right now," I said, "But I want you to know that when you're ready to, you can speak with one of us on the staff about it, to see how your feelings might fit in with your nervousness. In the meanwhile, we've got a number of different ways of helping with the nervousness and scared feelings you've been having. One possibility would be to stay here in the evening and at night when you've been having most of your trouble. Then you could go to work from here in the daytime."

We never did get to the other options, as the now surprised and surprising patient preempted the design of her own treatment plan with a question. "Well, can I go in now? My manager said to come back as soon as I can and if I hurry I can be there on time today." There was a brief discussion about possible use of medication, after which she got dressed and emerged in ten minutes with a smile on her face and an apron on her arm.

We had met our second lid man, and she was a woman. She told Dr. Sebastian that she was afraid to take medication because it might slow her down at work, but asked if she could see him later in the day after work. During their meetings in the next week she was able to speak about her recent parting with her boyfriend, and other periods in her life when she was harassed by persecutory voices. She readily agreed to follow-up visits with him after her discharge at the end of the week.

We returned to our coffee after that first meeting, and Joe said: "I can't believe what I just saw. If you had asked me to name one patient who wouldn't be going out of here on her own today she would have been the one. We were writing her up for direct transfer to St. Elizabeth's because she seemed so bogged down in the psychotic process. Then you began to talk with her in what had to be the most boring conversation of the year and I think to myself, Dr. Ryan has lost it. He's been working here too long. Now he's stuck in front of that cosmetics counter and he's never going to get out. And then all of a sudden I realized, hey, she's really getting turned on by that place. And the next thing you know, she's telling you all about her craziness, only she seems to be less afraid of the whole thing, like she's getting on your side and studying it a little. And then you talk with her about being a nighttime patient and I ask myself why didn't I think of that? Only I know why I didn't. She was just too far out of it." He paused and thought for a minute. "Now I have a feeling it's going to be all right for her to go to work today. In fact it would be the best treatment she could have. But how did you know she was going to be able to leave here like that?"

His invitation to indulge in a delusion of my omniscience was almost too much to resist. "She was obviously thinking about her work enough to tell the nurses about it," I replied, "so I put that down in my mind as a likely toehold in reality, and a good place for us to visit in for awhile. When she told me she had been there for seventeen years, I knew she had both feet firmly planted in the reality of her job. But the important happening was that we had something in common. She indeed valued her work, and I understood this aspect of herself and registered my approval. I let her know that I respected her and valued her for having this investment in her work. So I wasn't one of the "enemy out there" any longer. I'd gotten myself into the orbit of her self-love. As they say in the marketplace, "We had some good vibes going in both directions." And this was all that was necessary to rescue her from an empty, friendless and rage-filled world, even though most of the rage was of her own making."

"Wait a minute, Doc," said Walt, "You're going too fast for me. Where did you get that business about rage? She did look kind of hostile, and she was acting like she didn't want to have anything to do with anybody, but I don't see the rage in her. She was preoccupied with sex, not rage."

"All right, you've got me there. I'll have to admit I did some jumping to get to that conclusion. I've been thinking lately that it's the raw human destructive drives that set off the illness we call schizophrenia. I find myself at odds with Freud who said it was the sexual drives, in his paper on the Schreber case. I was making a guess when I brought in the idea of rage, but then look at it this way. Remember what Shakespeare said. He was the greatest psychiatrist of all. "Hell hath no fury like a woman scorned". I'm guessing that in the breakup she told us about she was probably jilted, and that she was dealing with the kind of fury Shakespeare referred to. In that case she might have withdrawn from everyone and from the world to keep the fury and rage from coming out in an overwhelming and harmful fashion. And this could be why she got mixed up about her sexual orientation. We'll find out more about this from her as we go along."

Joe and Walt caught the implications of this case immediately. Walt said, "We really shouldn't be sending anyone off to St. E's right away anymore", and Joe added "Amen". All of us were learning not to judge a book by its cover.

I looked forward to rounds later in the day, so that I could tell the group about our new rapid recovery patient. At the same time I had a vague sense of dissatisfaction with our previous discussions about the warming point. Something was missing. My voice of conscience intervened with a resounding "You dope. You forgot to make a connection with Freud's idea of a part of the schizophrenic that remained in touch with reality." The troubled woman we had just seen was a classic example of his important point. She might well have gone to St. Elizabeth's but for the fact that her job interest had been resistant to the schizophrenic process.

Applying Freud to the warming point it became clear that I had been probing for this island of rationality with every patient seen on rounds. The lid man was another good example of how this worked. Just before his plunge into overwhelming psychosis and word salad speech, his main reality interest had been to get himself into a hospital to guard against his rage harming others. His clenched jaw, rippling masseters and urge to run away reminded me of this, and his slip of the tongue about the lid put me right in touch with this real world concern. With both the lid man and the counter waitress I had been able to place myself right in the pathway of their principal concern in the real world. In consequence of this I was no longer a mechanical object "out there" but I became a real person. And so did the patient. We could begin to participate in the supportive and strengthening human interaction of sharing our inner warmth.

I told the rounds group that I had seen a new patient that morning, who had made such a rapid recovery that unfortunately she was no longer around to be interviewed. They laughed, and we settled down to a long discussion of the new patient, the warming point and Freud. At the end it was agreed that we still had considerably more to learn about the warming point.

6

Sharing inner warmth with delusional schizophrenics

After the discovery of the warming point there was still a danger of violence at D.C.General coming chiefly from two kinds of schizophrenics, the White House cases who were paranoid schizophrenics, and catatonic schizophrenics who were potentially homicidal. Rosie Gibson and Chris Welch, who was now a happily married Mrs. Goldhammer, each played a major role in reaching a warming point with them. In Rosie's case it happened one morning while we were discussing the Springtime arrival of so many visitors from around the country. Several of us were having coffee and talking about the good spirits of our tourists when Rosie reminded us of the one group of visitors who were very unhappy to be here, the White House cases. On our way upstairs from the coffee gathering, and with considerable hesitation, she told me she had a question to ask. "Dr. Ryan", she began, "would it be all right if we kept a pack of cigarettes on the nursing station for the White House people? They're all heavy smokers, and when they get here they don't have any cigarettes or money because the police take all of their possessions." There was a moment of silence on my part since we didn't encourage smoking and were trying to reduce the amount already done in the dayroom. Rosie went on, "You know, they all have nicotine stains on their fingers and some of them have the shakes from nicotine withdrawal." She had stated the plight of our White House cases with a humanity and concern that had been lacking in the rest of us. I said, "You're absolutely right. What good does it do to try to protect the future health of our patients when they're ready to explode right now from the shear frustration of being here. Go ahead, let's do it." The new nursing policy went into effect right away as she produced a fresh pack of cigarettes from her pocket.

Two days later I entered my own ward with the rounds group to see our latest arrival from the White House. He glowered at us as we drew near and motioned for us to go away with the wave of a very shaky hand. I said, "Good morning. Can I get you a cigarette? We have a pack on the nursing station." There was an instant warming point, indeed a ten, as he stammered a breathless "Y—Yes. Yes. Thank you." As he puffed on his cigarette we talked about his favorite brands, and then about getting his property back from the police. He told us all about his harassment by a group of unknown enemies with a degree of detachment, and finally concluded it had been foolish to try to get the president's help, because he was such a busy man. He was able to return home to New York with his brother on the next day.

This one case opened the way to a whole new approach towards the White House patients based on the simple sharing of our inner warmth with them right at the outset. Rosie Gibson had identified their most important real world interest that had not been touched by the schizophrenic withdrawal of these men. Tobacco craving was the first problem to be solved by doctor and patient together, and here indeed was a royal road to the warming point. It was remarkable. Their transition from a hostile or flat mood to one of warmth was every bit as abrupt and notable as it had been with the "lid man."

By providing cigarettes and talking with these patients about how we could recover their property, without even mentioning the White House, we soon found they would speak freely about their miserable lives in the grip of their delusions. We could agree with them that they had been suffering greatly, thus increasing the good human support and warmth we had to offer. It wasn't necessary to challenge the actual content of their false beliefs. We could accomplish more by simply listening. In time, and at their own pace, they could be expected to distance themselves from these firmly entrenched ideas, or at least diminish the impact of delusions on their lives.

We were learning an awful lot about treatment in a short time. The "lid man" was now succeeded by a whole new class of patients with whom we were able to share our inner warmth and modify the rage that had brought them to the White House. No longer a hostile nuisance, these men had become an inspiration. We were hot on the trail of a psychological explanation for schizophrenia.

In the lid man's case it was obvious that his illness had been driven by an upsurge in a particular instinctual drive—the urge to kill. It might have resulted in one of those tragic and inexplicable murders of several persons but for his lingering perception of this danger. These White House men had also harbored a great deal of hostility towards other humans as our staff had learned through many confrontations with their smoldering rage. We were now prepared to say that the clinical course of paranoid schizophrenia was determined by an abnormal overload of "raw destructive instinctual impulses" in a person.

These words are a psychiatrist's way of describing the part of our human nature that is most abhorrent to all of us, and also most disturbing. It is the residue of survival tactics that were necessary in mans earliest days on earth. We recognize the existence of these instincts most readily when we see them operating in others, as in ethnic wars or urban violence. But the urge to kill lies deeply buried in all of us, having been modified in varying degrees by experiencing the love of parents and others. The word "raw" touches on the fact that a portion of these instinctual urges may not be so well modified and can create an impetus to act with violence.

The White House patients had been blessed with high IQ's that they used to create elaborate systems of thought to explain why they were constantly at war with enemies. For awhile, this jerrybuilt defensive structure had allowed them to live marginal lives outside the hospital. Then something, some incident perhaps, or some chemical event in the brain, had increased the pressure from their destructive drives, making their symptoms unbearable. Only the most powerful man in the country could rescue them, and so they came to Washington to seek out the president. By this time their chronic low-grade withdrawal from the world had deepened and they needed human warmth (loving energies) from others to offset and tame their destructive impulses. In the warming point they received the very first dose of this healing medicine.

Catatonic patients who were mute and immobile were still the greatest menace to the rest of the community. They were using the last ditch defenses of keeping a total watch on their surroundings and themselves, and clamping a tight hold on their musculature to stifle a powerful urge to commit mass murder.

One morning I had an emergency call from Mrs. Goldhammer, who was not given to making such calls. "Can you come up here and give us a hand?" she asked. "We've got a man who looks like he's about to blow, and I haven't been able to reach Miss Shea to get some more men up here." When I arrived on the ward, I could see just what she meant. In the center of the dayroom stood a tall, muscular young man, his body erect and rigid, with jaw protruding and gaze set straight ahead. He could have been made of stone, his face chiseled into a fixed expression of pain. The only sign of life was a tear that had developed in the corner of one eye, and coursed silently over a frozen cheek. He did in fact look like a statue—a living monument to the mentally ill.

I had seen any number of men in a crisis like that before, but on this particular morning it really got to me. Maybe it was the frightened look in Chris's eyes—or watching Alston and Gerry circle the dayroom, pretending involvement in other chores, but walking on eggshells lest they disturb the man of stone. They were in the mode of maximal alertness, ready to attempt a two-man tackle if necessary, but knowing their quarry might be in the mode to kill. "God help that poor man" I thought, and "God help the rest of us if he goes on a rampage."

Putting on our best looks of quiet professional concern, Chris and I approached him. We had recently been talking about the best way to greet catatonics who were mute, and had agreed it was important not to make a demand on them for speech. "Eddie", she said simply, "This is Dr. Ryan and he wants to help you."

Addressing him as softly as possible I said, "I know that you can't speak right now but that you can hear me. You look like you've been having a lot of pain and I want to help you. You'll be able to speak again, and when you can, I'll come back. Just let one of the staff know, and they'll call me."

As we started away, he attempted to speak. At first only the letter "S" could come, but soon, in repetitive form, it was SSSS_SSSS_SSSS." Was he hissing like a snake to warn us away? Or was he struggling with a very difficult topic? Words finally emerged : "My SSS—SSS—sister is getting married. But she's inside me and so is my mother. My heart has broken into pieces and it can't keep them alive much longer."

He was trying to tell us of the heavy burden that had been placed on his heart by his sister's wedding plans. As he rambled on about the workings of his shattered heart, his thinking was still in a psychotic vein. I was troubled by how little connection I felt between us, and had to remind myself of the cardinal rule: Keep listening to what the patient has to say. It became clear that he was struggling with many questions about his family: "Where were they? What were they doing? Were they even alive?

The opportunity for a sharing of inner warmth was at hand. "Shall we call them now?" I asked pleasantly, "to see what they're up to?"

"That would be wonderful," he replied, with a sudden happiness that seemed to know no bounds.

We retreated to the nursing station where he had trouble dialing the number and asked me in a halting voice to do it for him. He took the phone with trembling hands and a woman's voice answered "Hello". Eddie shouted a breathless "Mom! Is that you? Are you all right?"

"Of course I am", she answered matter of factly. She quickly added, "You sound upset. Are you okay? Where are you?" "I'm in the D.C.General Hospital, and"

His mother's voice cut him short. "Oh my God," she said, "something terrible has happened. What is it? I'll come right over." They lived on nearby Capitol Hill.

There was a peaceful expression on Eddie's face before his response, that disappeared as he started to speak. "I'm, I'm feeling strange mom. SS Something is happening to me. I'm scared. My body is getting tight all over." He paused as if straining to get out the next words. The peaceful look had been replaced by a troubled scowl, and I feared the worst. He was slipping into a catatonic state right before our eyes.

"My heart. My h-h-heart," he resumed.

His mother cut in again. "Which part of the hospital are you in? Give me some directions."

Eddie stood there silently, looking somewhat dazed while Chris got on the line and provided directions. After the call he appeared to forget about the broken heart and endangered family members within himself. His most retained interest in the real world had been his mother, and by joining him there we had helped him to turn away from the psychotic creatures inside himself to the real mother and sister who were alive and well at home. In the process, we too, had become flesh and blood people for him, and Eddie himself felt like a real human being again.

Eddie's mother and sister came over within an hour of the telephone call. While his mother was visiting with him, his sister provided some valuable background information. Eddie had in fact been born with a "broken" heart, that is to say a large defect in the septum that separated the two auricular chambers. The murmur created by this hole in one of the inner cardiac walls was so loud that they could hear it as they stood by his crib. His parents had been told that the defect should become smaller over the next several months, and might even close completely in time. Meanwhile there was nothing that could be done about it, and they would simply have to be very watchful and bring him into the emergency room if they saw any sign of distress.

His mother had been distraught at the news and she spoke of her baby's "broken heart" to almost anyone she might meet. She picked him up constantly, holding him next to her own heart, and she wouldn't permit anyone else to touch him, including his father. The latter had been disturbed by his wife's behavior and tried to console himself by heavy drinking. At the end of his son's first year he succumbed to a sudden death due to a heart attack.

To his sister's best knowledge Eddie's cardiac defect had closed by age two or three, but his mother remained fiercely protective of her "baby". Eddie was kept indoors and not allowed to play with other youngsters. For the first six grades, his mother had escorted him to and from school every day. By the seventh he was travelling there alone but had to give his mother a full account of his whereabouts if he did not return home directly. It was pretty much the same in high school, but that was all right; he was inclined to come home anyway because he had so few friends. He attended a local college where, as before, he had few friends and lived at home. After college he got a job as a teller in a nearby bank, sometimes returning home for lunch. His mother selected all his clothing, bought the groceries and cooked supper for his sister and himself. He had never shown any desire to move away from home.

His sister acknowledged that she too had been protective of her brother and didn't seem to think her mother's behavior unusual. She characterized their family as "very, very close." She recognized that her plans to marry had caused her brother considerable grief. He was intensely jealous of all the time his mother was now devoting to making arrangements for the wedding.

"Several weeks ago", she said, "Eddie began to sulk and mutter complaints under his breath." Then he started carrying on conversations with himself. A few days before his hospital admission, he berated his mother in unusually harsh and hostile tones, causing her great alarm. His sister had suggested they bring him to D.C.General for psychiatric evaluation but his mother bristled at this idea. She denied that he had a mental illness and feared that "They might try to put him in St. Elizabeth's for a long time."

It seemed clear that Eddie had been caught up in a symbiotic relationship with his mother, and virtually depended on the maternal heartbeat for his survival. His sister's plans for marriage were now threatening both the breakup of their "very, very close" family, and more immediately, his vital dependency on his mother. Such a severe blow to his whole sense of what was right and just in the world, and necessary for his very life, was bound to stir up an enormous amount of primitive rage.

There were no more episodes of muteness or catatonia. The restoration of loving contact with his mother and sister had tamed his rage and started a healing process. But that process still had a long way to go.

Eddie needed help escaping the destructive bond he had forged with his mother. To jump-start this phase of his treatment, he was moved from the locked confines of Unit Eight to the small open ward on the second floor. Here he had his own room and lived away from home for the first time in his life, learning to function on his own. He liked the young resident doctor who was assigned to his case and began to model himself after this man, even buying a sport jacket quite similar to his doctor's. With the latter's help he contacted some of his former college classmates and managed to find places to go with them. Eddie had to overcome a shyness and social withdrawal of major dimensions, but he made it. After a few months on the open ward he moved into a rented home with three other young men who also were recent college graduates.

Eddie's treatment wasn't as easy as its brevity and successful outcome might suggest. He was on fairly heavy doses of Thorazine during the first three weeks because this was the standard treatment for so highly dangerous an illness as catatonic schizophrenia. The daily visits with his family were helpful but always followed by relapses into states of withdrawal, flat affect and occasional auditory hallucinations. It was only after a reduction of his Thorazine dosage that he began slowly, and cautiously to relate to his resident therapist. Even as they got to know each better he experienced episodes of suspicion and mistrust. For his therapist, yesterday's progress was often today's disappointment and tomorrow's anxious uncertainty. The slow march to the dominance of rationality was equally tedious for his family, but in the end, Eddie emerged as a new person, stronger and more capable of sharing his own warmth with others than before.

He wasn't free of the danger of relapse, and probably never will be. Schizophrenia is a tenacious illness, which is embedded in the genes and may come back. But Eddie could now make friends and enjoy their company. He was also dating women for the first time in his life. Could he marry and raise a family? Quite possibly, only time would tell.

The case of Mr. Edward A. was a wonderful tonic for an ailing hospital that was only starting on the road to recovery and new life. It confirmed our belief that schizophrenia was not a hopeless disease, not a medical monster that required long term custody in the hope it might eventually wear itself out. It pointed the way to a new approach to schizophrenic treatment. Under the old system, still the existing system, catatonic schizophrenia mandated radical treatment. In other local hospitals such patients were placed in "cold packs", tied down in bed swathed in sheets filled with ice, presumably to cool the violence burning within. If agitated, they were placed in tubs of warm water covered by a canvas bonnet that allowed only their heads to protrude. The treatment of choice was electroshock, subjecting their bodies to violent convulsions in the hope of discharging their rage.

We now had something new to offer, getting through with inner warmth. It was a specific therapy, that is it involved introducing a therapeutic agent, human warmth, into the patient, as a specific antidote for the pathologic process, an overload of the destructive drives. Obviously the sooner this could be done the better. The "lid man", counter waitress, White House cases, and a catatonic schizophrenic in crisis had taught us this could be done in a first meeting. Could it always be done that way? Based on our past deeply entrenched convictions about the difficulty of treating schizophrenics, most of us were not yet that optimistic. It was a treatment experience that required steady repetition. How to do this in a busy acute receiving hospital was another question. We were convinced that the old system was wrong but we didn't exactly know how to fix it.

7

Mourning and the roots of the warming point

At this juncture in my narrative of the progress made at D.C.General it seems appropriate to talk about where my powerful wish to converse rationally with schizophrenics was coming from. That belated insight came to me only after writing the full story. The secret of what made the sharing of inner warmth with schizophrenics possible was finally clear. I was busily engaged in a healing of myself.

By far the most traumatic experience in my life was my mother's death. It was no ordinary death since she was murdered in the course of a violent rape, about three years before my discovery of the warming point. She was a healer who had given up her profession as a nurse to lovingly raise five children. She often had other children or young adults stay with us in their hour of need, and had a circle of friends who called her regularly on the telephone for help. She was killed on her way to a night meeting for a charitable cause.

The terrible news came to me in a phone call at three in the morning. I cried until dawn when I made my way to Union Station for a train to New York. How could my mother, a woman of such goodness, become the brutalized victim of a terrible crime? My pain was intense, and everything in the outside world was suddenly painful too, because it reminded me of my overwhelming loss. My mother's murder made headline news in New York, making the walk through Penn Station a searing torture. There was outrage as well as pain, but the pain muted the outrage into a periodic awareness of the phrase "a crime that cries out to heaven for vengeance."

When I got home I was preoccupied with trying to ease my father's agony. He had depended on my mother to manage his diabetes, and to lay out his entire day's wardrobe each morning. My sister and three brothers were already there, and we shared our hugs and tears with my father. As we reviewed the horrible events of the night before, a new question emerged. What were we to tell my mother's five grandchildren? How were we to explain her death to them? She had been the kind of adoring grandmother who always had some special present for each one on their weekly visits, and they loved her intensely. It would be a devastating introduction to human brutality no matter how we presented it. We agreed to tell them the basic truth that she had been killed instantly by an unknown man who struck her on the head with a rock. They were also to be told that Uncle Jim had said that a man who would do something terrible like that is usually out of his mind and suffering from a serious mental illness. Our worry over the children's loss provided a momentary distraction from our own severe pain and gave us a good topic to focus on. We had all taken on my mother's role of healer.

The tremendous number of people who trooped through the funeral home to share their warmth helped us enormously at the wake. They came from every borough and every suburb, each offering fond memories of what a beautiful person my mother was. New York City became a warm and friendly village in that packed mortuary. Classmates from grade school, Regis High, college, med school, and even people I was meeting for the first time were able to get through with loving feelings to replenish our family's damaged supply.

When we took our seats in the limousine behind the hearse I had a strange and meaningful experience. To accommodate all of us I had to sit in the front seat next to the driver, and was separated from my family by a glass panel. The driver himself was standing outside and my own window was securely locked. As I looked ahead at my mother's coffin, and then at passersby, I suddenly felt very cold and very small. I thought to myself, "Those people outside are so large and full of life, and I feel like a little five-year-old." And then I thought of my mother and myself when I was actually five years old. We were seated on a couch in the living room, next to each other, and she was holding an open missal, showing me the Latin phrases used in the Mass. I began to cry, out of an admixture of sadness and joy. The greatest accomplishment of my early life had been to become an altar boy at five so that I could serve Mass with my older brother. My mother had made this possible by helping me to meet the requirement of knowing all the Latin responses in the Mass.

With the help of his children and friends, my father recovered from a state of abject despair in about a year. One day, shortly thereafter, he announced to a group of former business associates that he was "feeling so young again" that he was going to come out of retirement to help expand our family's business. That very evening, he sat back in his favorite chair, dozed off briefly, and succumbed to a sudden death coronary occlusion. So the violent attack of a murderer, who I guessed was probably a schizophrenic, had taken a second life.

I was only getting along marginally well towards the end of that year, and one evening I confided to a friend that I was "leading a dog's life." For several months I had not been doing my best work at the hospital, and had accumulated a backlog of court cases that included murderers and rapists. I had stubbornly refused the Chief Psychiatrist's offer to divert them from me, but I was staggering under the total load. My part-time private practice had also become too busy and demanding, and my avocation as a night law student at the Georgetown University Law School was another source of great fatigue. I wasn't aware that the greatest weight on my shoulders was the still unresolved residue of rage from my mother's violent death. My father's death reopened that wound and added a new layer of pain.

My mother's death had occurred only nine months after the start of my career as a forensic psychiatrist. The irony of the task of gaining intimate knowledge about murderers weighed heavily on me in those early days after her murder. I didn't want to see any such individuals and took advantage of the ninety day commitment periods to postpone first interviews as long as possible. Chief Judge David Bazelon, of the U.S. Court of Appeals for the D.C. Circuit, had sternly objected to the brevity of my evaluations in one of his opinions. His criticism, as it turned out, was totally justified, but I was too wiped out emotionally to do anything constructive about it. Later, as my healing progressed and my appetite for court work returned, I was invited into the Yale Law School study of the Durham Rule by the lead attorney, Richard Arens. By spending at least twenty hours in each evaluation, instead of the usual two there was a natural progression into a doctor-patient relationship with a sharing of inner warmth. Defendants who had previously denied any mental problems began to open up and reveal psychotic conditions that had been present at the time of their crimes. As the study went on, we found more and more such individuals and arrived at the conclusion that a great many murders and violent rapes are directly caused by schizophrenic illnesses that remain undetected due to inadequate psychiatric evaluation. I presented these findings in a paper delivered at the annual meeting of the American Psychiatric Association in my home city of New York in May 1963. My mother and father were no longer around to hear or read this paper. The sure knowledge they would have been proud of me was another step in healing myself.

The most important ingredient in my healing came about by pure chance, (or more likely by the intervention of my mother's soul), on the same day I had complained about "leading a dog's life." I was a very tired dog on that particular evening and had decided not to go to the second of three going-away parties being held for a lawyer friend, Bill Cooney. Stretching out in the interns' quarters for a brief rest before my law school class my bones ached and my eyes throbbed. I congratulated myself on the decision to skip the party. Then, suddenly, I was struck by the thought, "I can't stay away from Bill's party tonight. He's my good friend. I'll go very early, and if I'm too tired, I'll just leave early."

My plan led me to be the first guest to arrive and allowed me to trade some stories with Bill while our hosts scurried about getting ready to greet the large number expected at their door. One of the first arrivals was a young married couple, who were accompanied by a girl with a beautifully warm smile—obviously the wife's younger sister. That smile radiated across the room to touch my heart, quicken circulation and banish fatigue. It was an instant getting through with inner warmth. "Bill, that smile", I said, "I've got to meet her", and we became the first to greet the threesome.

It turned out that the younger woman, whose name was Priscilla, had also come early anticipating a short stay. She was in town for a three day visit with her sister and would return on Sunday to Pittsburgh to complete her senior year at Mt. Mercy College. We both stayed at the party much later than expected, and were almost always together, even while we talked with other guests. It was a wonderful start to a courtship that led to our engagement at Christmastime and marriage in early May. As we visited back and forth across the country, I soon learned that prolonged exposure to Priscilla's engaging smile and warm heart had cured my "dog's life" syndrome, and created a new enthusiasm in me for both court case examinations and nighttime law school. Heavy fatigue was no longer a problem.

The significance of my recovery from such disabling states of fatigue can be briefly summarized, love had won out over hate. I had been blessed with a massive increase in loving energies from the steady exchange of love with my fiancée. The healing power of unselfish love had been able to tame the powerful rage and sense of injustice caused by my mother's murder. The extra expenditure of energy needed to control rage was no longer required, and could be put into creative new uses. The discovery of the warming point in schizophrenia was one of these, and some insights into schizophrenia as a cause of criminal behavior was another.

A tragic loss cannot be undone, but the wounded survivor is almost always strengthened by the adoption of some of the deceased's best ways through identification (achieving a personality makeover by becoming like the deceased.) We hold on to the departed object of our love by taking in some of his or her personality traits and remodeling ourselves to reflect these features. This taking in of my mother opened the door to powerful new life interests and accomplishments that hastened the overcoming of the traumatic event.

My sudden and unexpected zeal to hold rational conversations with the deeply psychotic had an explanation. It was the wonderful mother of my fifth year who had encouraged me to look at the strange language of Latin, and told me I could read it, understand it, memorize it and become an altar boy. The image of a caring mother in interaction with a little boy had become a permanent part of my memory, built into me for future use. The mother was in fact reassuring that little boy that he could do something special with his mind during times when she was busy with his three younger siblings. Thus it had been born out of many moments of painful loss when she had had her hands full in the service of three younger rivals for her love. Now in the days of greatest loss the power of that image to heal had survived, and was again moving my psyche in new directions.

The shocking loss of a murdered mother had reawakened the healing and sustaining inner presence of the mother of my fifth year. She was urging me to find a way to speak and share some warmth with patients who were struggling with the most overwhelming and inhuman kinds of destructive drive pressures. Her clear message was that I had something good inside myself that could help to sooth these raw destructive energies in others who were so overwhelmed by them that they had been forced to withdraw entirely from the world. I'm sure too, in the very back of my mind, and out of conscious awareness, was the notion that she would have wanted me to find out more about the malignant forces that could have caused someone to kill her.

Healing of the self is a lifetime effort because there are so many events that can stir up our rage. The experience of mourning is something we all must go through at one time or another. My mother's death was acutely traumatic because it was totally unexpected and involved a crushing blow to my own sense of what was right and just in the world. The presence of overpowering rage revealed itself in two forms, intense pain alternating with numbness. The driving force of emotional pain is rage turned against the self to protect against the danger of losing control over the outward release of rage. Numbness, performing life's tasks like a robot, serves the same purposes. Edward Bibring, M.D. made this point beautifully in his paper on depression when he called the reaction of depersonalization "a last ditch defense of the ego against overwhelming rage." It is the final way station of normalcy before the total shutdown of feelings that occurs in schizophrenia, or causes the inability to move seen in hysterical paralysis on the battlefield.

Numbness was there in moments of solitude but it gave way to sharing warmth with family and friends whenever they were around. Healing was enhanced by allowing a flood of memories of my mother to flow over me, in a frantic effort to hold on to her and deny her death, even while extracting a further supply of loving energies to cope with rage. The mourning process takes a long time because the loss of someone really close continues to generate rage until it can finally gain acceptance. The sense that I was "leading a dog's life" ten months after my mother's death and suffering from unaccustomed fatigue were signs of unmetabolized rage. Eventually, I was able to accept the tragic loss with the help of my love for Priscilla, and her love for me.

My technique for working with schizophrenics was best summarized by my friend and colleague, Dr. Jerry Styrt of Baltimore, with whom I taught the course in schizophrenia at the Baltimore-Washington Institute for Psychoanalysis. One evening after class, he said "I've been trying to think why you've had so much success with schizophrenics. I used to think it was because you were so comfortable with being the object of a maternal transference, but I think it's something much more. There is a spiritual quality to your work with them." I believe he was right. It was the spirit of my mother working within me, and guiding me on how to get through to them with inner warmth.

8

D.C. General, under new management

It was a wonderful time, a strange time and a frustrating time in my life as a psychiatrist. Many months had passed since the discovery of the warming point, but the only sign of progress in our work was a reduction in the number of White House cases awaiting their transfer to St. Elizabeth's. If anything we were moving the other patients through the revolving door more rapidly. That was due in part to the superb administrative skills of John Schultz's successor as Chief Psychiatrist, Dr. Mary MacIndoo.

I liked Mary. She had been kind and helpful to me at the time of my mother's death even though she usually kept her personal warmth to herself. Her trademark was her long silver cigarette holder that she used to flick her ash in disdain should someone disagree with her. She wasn't psychoanalytically minded but she used her good knowledge of classical psychiatry to run the hospital more efficiently and effectively than John Schultz. In other words she was making the old system work at its best and there was no indication that this might change on the horizon. She appeared to like her job, but one day she surprised us all and announced that she had accepted a new position at the VA down South. Her successor was the Associate Chief Psychiatrist, Dr. Jim Foy, who in turn named me to his old job. It was a day of liberation for both of us and opened the way to the remodeling of our program.

A fresh breeze was soon blowing across D.C.General and it was issuing forth from the office of the new Chief Psychiatrist, Dr. Jim Foy. Unlike his two predecessors, whose strengths were administration, Jim was primarily a teacher and an intellectual. He had been hired by Georgetown to run the academic program for students at D.C.General, his only other task being to supervise the open ward. In this capacity he had promoted a more psychologically minded approach to both illness and patient care throughout the hospital, and his personal warmth as Chief made for better staff morale. More than anything he had helped to foster a new spirit of inquiry into many aspects of our work.

One of our areas of mutual interest had to do with the forensic psychiatric examinations now being conducted by the entire staff under the Durham Rule for the insanity defense. I had given a paper on this subject at the annual meeting of the American Psychiatric Association in May of 1963, and Jim differed strongly with one of the conclusions. The paper dealt with several cases in which there was clear evidence of schizophrenic illness at the time of the crime that had gone undetected by other psychiatrists who testified at the trial. Since my own findings had come only after many hours of interview time, I had suspected that routine psychiatric examinations with negative results might be failing to uncover serious disturbances at the time of the crime. Jim challenged this notion thinking that I had come upon a few exceptional cases in which the other experts hadn't done their work. He was sure that a well-qualified psychiatrist would almost always be able to find some evidence of a recent psychotic condition.

One Monday morning, about a year after Jim's promotion, I arrived on the ward to find that a famous Durham Rule criminal had been admitted the night before for mental observation. A policeman had seen him walking down the middle of a busy Washington street, mumbling about voices and apparently oblivious to the danger of passing cars. He was not charged with any crime. His status of mental observation meant that we had to study his behavior in the hospital and refer him to the Mental Health Commission for commitment to St. Elizabeth's if we found him to be suffering from a mental illness dangerous to himself or others. My pulse quickened at the prospect of meeting him for the first time. He had been examined by so many psychiatrists, and with such conflicting opinions that I was eager to join the fray. I knew that Jim would want to see him also, since the patient's case was one of a small group of Durham Rule cases under intense scrutiny by the psychiatric and legal professions.

Entering his bedroom I found a young man seated on his bed, staring blankly into space and conversing in a totally flat way with imaginary voices. I tried to engage him in a conversation of some kind without success. He was completely withdrawn from the world with the most classic example of flat affect that I had encountered in many months. I hastened to call Jim Foy and found him as excited as I had been to have this man in our hospital. "I'll be right up", he said, and in moments he was trying as vainly as I to make contact with our patient. He too was impressed with his profound flatness of affect and said, "Well, there's no doubt about this diagnosis. He's an unquestioned schizophrenic and from that affect he looks like he might have been in this state for some time." For both of us it was a historic moment because we knew that he hadn't presented with a clear-cut diagnosis of schizophrenia during a number of previous hospitalizations and psychiatric examinations.

At this point I had an inspiration. It was at a time when we were beginning to see rapid recoveries in many of our psychotic patients as a result of the discovery of the warming point. Neither Jim nor I had been able to reach one with him, but I reminded Jim that our nursing assistants had been increasingly successful in sharing their inner warmth with psychotic patients and bringing them out of this state in a few days. I said, "I wouldn't be a bit surprised if he had reverted to his normal personality, which I presume is sociopathic, by Thursday of this week. If that happens we could ask Bill Novak, who was in charge of our residency program, to do a one hour forensic evaluation of him in his conference with the residents on Thursday. I'll keep his chart and we won't provide him with any information about his condition on admission. We'll tell Bill that we might have to answer the Durham Rule question about whether he had any illness during the week or month before his admission, and so to be on the lookout for any evidence of a schizophrenic condition. Then we'll meet him after the conference to get his opinion."

Jim laughed and said, "You don't give up, do you? If he's that much better we'll do it, and I'll bet you Bill will have a lot to say about his schizophrenia."

"O.K.," said I, "It's a bet. And if he's not ready this Thursday I'm sure we can do it on the next one."

When Thursday rolled around I pronounced our patient ready for the test, and Bill conducted a very thorough evaluation before the assembled residents. He was one of our best examiners with a solid background of psychoanalytic training. Jim and I descended on him immediately afterward with, "Well, what did you find?"

"He's a sociopath all right, pure and simple," Bill said. "A classic case and a good one to present to the residents."

"Well, did you see any residuals of schizophrenia or anything that might make you suspect he was one before he came in?" asked Jim. "Not a trace," said Bill. "I asked him how he was doing those last couple of weeks and he said "I was fine. I was working on my house." Like I said, "He's a sociopath, pure and simple."

Jim and I broke out in laughter and let Bill in on the joke. He was not amused at first, and then he too laughed and said, "Well, that's a sociopath for you. They're very good at hiding what they don't want you to know."

Both of them turned to me and said, "What made you think he would get better so quickly?"

I replied, "Well, I don't know. I guess I just had an intuitive feeling about it."

"There you go again, you and your intuition" was their rejoinder. What I didn't tell them was that my intuition was bolstered by recent experiences with dramatic schizophrenic reversals that I was still finding hard to believe.

We began then to take a more serious look at the clinical event we had just witnessed. Once again one of our patients had made a rapid recovery from an acute schizophrenic illness. Jim and I were adamant about the diagnosis based on the profound disturbance of affect we had seen. It couldn't possibly have been faked. The three of us were willing to consider the term "schizophreniform disorder" recently introduced to cover persons with very brief episodes of illness, but my colleagues still wanted to know if there had been a turning point.

I said, "There had. It was in the evening shift on Monday when David Jerry came on duty. The patient had been reclusive and hallucinating all day long but he heard Jerry talking with another patient about the Orioles game that day. Somehow he and Jerry got into a conversation about the team and it turned out both of them were rabid Orioles fans. After that he got into a discussion about baseball with some other patients, and he seemed to be pretty rational from then on. Next morning he asked when Jerry would be coming and they've spent some time together every day since." It looked like another instance in which there had been a warming point and a turning point, and we agreed that we were beginning to have a more hopeful attitude about schizophrenia.

The three of us were the same age and had the benefit of the same kind of training that was fostering a new generation of optimistic psychiatrists. We were also the three senior psychiatrists in the building by now and shared the responsibility of helping the med students and residents to think in more positive ways about mental illness. We took some time to consider how we might increase their awareness of the importance of good human contact, and Bill reported on a project he had just begun that looked like a promising teaching device.

He had been concerned for some time that the residents were placing too much reliance on Thorazine as though it were the only effective and therefore necessary treatment for schizophrenia. To improve their judgment about its use, and also to enhance their clinical appraisal of patients, he had begun declaring certain days to be drug free. On these days psychiatric medications were not to be ordered for new admissions unless absolutely necessary. This would allow for a twenty-four hour period in which to get to know patients better and see what could be accomplished without medication. He had already found that some patients could do better without drugs and reported that dosage levels of Thorazine had dropped in the building. Jim and I agreed that Bill had taken a bold and worthwhile step in the right direction.

The Jim Foy era was marked by another series of events that bore witness to his creativity and readiness to ask new questions. His favorite perk as Chief Psychiatrist was the control it gave him over the use of our Auditorium. He indulged this power in two notable ways. For one thing he founded a cinema club for the showing and discussion of art films, just before his promotion. The club now found a splendid new home and the movies inevitably dealt with important psychological issues, which gave rise to spirited discussion. The value of these well-attended meetings made us all feel better about our affiliation with D.C.General.

His daytime plans for the auditorium called for doctors who had already made notable contributions to psychiatry to speak. Two of these visitors had a very significant impact on our program. The first was Dr.Robert Knight, a physician and psychoanalyst, who headed one of the most highly regarded psychoanalytic treatment centers in the world, the Austen-Riggs Center in Stockbridge, Massachusetts. He offered a number of examples of how they were trying to give their patients a greater say in their own treatment. These had led to some major changes in their own operation. He also told some poignant stories about his closest colleague there, Dr. David Rappaport, from the months before his recent sudden death. Dr. Rappaport had been one of the leading American psychoanalysts and a frequent participant in meetings at the Beth Israel Hospital. For me, the whole afternoon evoked shades of Camelot.

Austen-Riggs had a large open ward where patients frequently made decisions that had to be cleared with the staff. As an example he told how he and Dr. Rappaport had to agonize over a request by their entertainment committee to serve alcoholic beverages at an upcoming reception. They came down on the side of upholding this request and were rewarded by the thoughtful safeguards that the committee developed for alcohol use at the event.

An even more meaningful speaker as things later turned out was Dr. Jack Ewalt, President of the American Psychoanalytic Association and Chief Psychiatrist at the Massachusetts Mental Health Center, Dr. Ewalt gave a dramatic and inspiring account of how they had transformed their hospital from a locked facility for mostly psychotic patients to one that was completely open. The most startling piece of information was his claim that there were no longer any overt schizo-phrenics in the building. He too provided lots of clinical data to back up this claim.

Dr. Ewalt had come to provide consultation on our program, as well as to give a talk about his own open hospital. He visited a number of wards and made suggestions as he went. At the end of the day, after his formal presentation, he announced that there was just time for one or two more questions. My hand was in the air before he even completed his words. "Dr. Ewalt, what do you think are the possibilities for D.C. General to become an open hospital?"

His answer was absolutely clear. "You couldn't possibly do that here!" He almost sounded a little insulted by the idea but he recovered his composure and gave the question serious consideration. "First of all, you just don't have the quality and depth of nursing staff that we do at Massachusetts Mental Health. Many of our nurses have masters degrees in psychiatric nursing and we have a much higher staff/patient ratio than you do. The second reason is that you have no control at all over your admissions. You're a public mental hospital and have to take in everyone who comes to your door. No matter how unruly or dangerous they may be. At least we can refuse certain patients if they do not fit in with our program." The day concluded with enthusiastic applause, my own included, for what had truly been a remarkable presentation.

I felt depressed after Dr. Ewalt's final comments and allowed his forceful answer to shut down my own speculation for a while. Not for long. He had struck a nerve with his words about our nursing staff, and I was in a fighting mood. "Where does he get off with that stuff about nurses with masters degrees? It's not what's in the head but what's in the heart that counts, and our staff is really strong in that department. Very strong." I thought of Leroy Alston and David Jerry and wasn't sure that either one had a high school degree. Chris Goldhammer and

Rosie Gibson certainly were not college graduates, nor was anyone else on our nursing staff except maybe Helen Shea. And yet these people had managed a floodtide of admissions for many years with no "certain patients" they could refuse. They were solid people, loyal and devoted to their work and showing a very steady increase in successful outcomes for their efforts.

All of these thoughts were still running through my mind prior to the next Monday staff meeting, but I didn't expect to speak there. Others would have much to say and I wanted to listen first. Then Jim Foy turned to me at the outset of the meeting and said, "Jim, what did you think about Dr. Ewalt's talk?" He opened a floodgate.

Everything I had just alluded to came out in a torrent of words and feelings, along with much more. I began to review experiences I had had over the years with so many of the nurses and nursing assistants by way of illustrating their exceptional character. I had never talked so long at any of our meetings, and was beginning to feel carried away by my own pressure of speech when suddenly I hit upon a new topic that had been on my mind for some time.

"Now there's one problem I think we're going to have to address right now because it's existed so long, and caused so much grief already, and that's the sexual integration of our wards. It's just not natural for men and women to live completely segregated from one another, and it shows a lack of respect for the members of both sexes to insist that they do so. Dr. Knight was right. We've got to show our patients that we trust in their ability to regulate their own behavior appropriately. If we don't do this then we are depriving them of some very critical input necessary for their recovery."

"We ought to talk about this some more next week and after that announce to all the patients that it's going to happen in one month, so that they'd have time to plan for whatever adjustments might be needed on each ward. Our patient-staff committees would have to work overtime, but I think they should be given a precise deadline for the changeover."

Having said all this, I realized that the main point in the back of my mind was just coming into focus, and so I presented it as an afterthought. "Once we have the units sexually integrated we ought to move ahead with a plan to unlock them, maybe allowing another two months to accomplish this step."

The room drew its collective breath at that point. Jim Foy had created a wonderful town meeting type of ambience for his staff meetings and so it was not unusual for one of us to bring up novel or controversial ideas just for feedback. Two of the members were already in a state of semi-shock, namely Paul Barnes and George Hall who ran the two female units.

Paul Barnes opened with, "Wait a minute. You've got some guys on the male side that you just can't put in with the women. You've got some criminals and even rapists. It wouldn't be safe. I suppose if you could lock those fellows up on the old maximum security court unit we might give it a try. We'd have to put the women on one end wing and the men on the other end wing, and keep the middle one open as a neutral zone." George Hall was equally concerned, and backed Paul on every point, including the neutral zone. They were already prepared for an outbreak of war between the sexes.

Helen Shea as usual had her finger on the pulse of the anxiety within Paul and George and she knew just what to do to tone it down. Turning to them with her warm smile she acknowledged their right to be worried, and said she was sure all of their nurses would be anxious too. She reminded all of us that we had had the most notorious serial rapist in modern D.C. history as a patient on the maximum security unit three years before, and that we had only been able to close that ward after his departure. By then St. Elizabeth's had completed construction of an even more secure facility for dangerous court referrals, so we were no longer getting court patients who provided an immediate risk to others.

She was prepared to address the topic of anxiety about rape with the nurses and patients of the female wards, and she was sure they could come to terms with their worries. She then made an interesting observation: "You know, I visit all the wards every day so naturally I do some comparing of one with another. The men are really much better behaved sexually and otherwise when women come on their unit, than the women are with male visitors. Some of the women are inclined to make crude sexual remarks towards men, or they shy away from them like they are intruders. I agree with Dr. Ryan. Men and women were really made to be around one another so I'm all for getting them together and I think one month gives us enough time." Mother Superior had spoken and given the integration plan her blessing. There was harmony in the room as the meeting ended.

Jim Foy looked like he had something on his mind, and asked if I could stay a few minutes afterward. The something proved to be a bombshell as far as I was concerned. He wanted to tell me that he would be leaving the job of Chief Psychiatrist in three weeks in order to occupy a new teaching position that had just been created at the Georgetown University Hospital. "So I'll be out of here long before the integration of the wards. They really wanted me to come in just two weeks but there's so much detail to be gone through here that I couldn't possibly have done that. I've recommended you for the Chief's position, and I'm hoping and praying that you'll take it. There's a lot of stress in this job but no more than you've had to deal with in the Court Service. Dick Steinbach, the Professor of Psychiatry at Georgetown, and John

Schultz both want you to be the Chief Psychiatrist so this office will be yours if you say "Yes."

I had expected Jim would be Chief for at least another five years, and I would be entering full time private practice in perhaps two, after he and I had completed the project of opening the hospital. I told him this and he laughed, saying that that might take a lot more years than two, but now I'd have to go it alone.

A period of sober thought followed because I really had been looking forward to working with Jim on the further development of our whole program. The plan I had just outlined would have been carried out by Jim with my assistance. In this scenario he was to execute, and I could sit back and enjoy the splendor of my ideas. But now the moment of truth had arrived. As the saying goes, I had to put my money where my mouth was. Could I really be in charge of a large organization? If I wanted to realize my dream I would have to assume more responsibility and work much harder than anticipated. Suddenly the question of obstacles to an open and sexually integrated hospital loomed into focus and I asked Jim for his reading on the whole thing.

"It won't be easy, that's for sure, but we can start with some pluses. The Central Nursing Office has eased up on us thanks to Helen Shea. Miss Ritter, (the D.C.G.H. Director of Nursing), has been coming over here more often because she likes what she is seeing. She was really pleased with your recommendation that Rosie Gibson and Chris Gold-hammer be given outstanding ratings, and she'll go along with any changes you suggest. The same is true of the Medical Director for different reasons. He has so much trouble on his hands from the rest of the hospital that he doesn't get into our operation at all."

Just between you and me I think the biggest problem is going to be the judges and prosecutors. They've been using us as a convenient place to take people off the streets who don't belong there. I don't think that's going to change. We're part of the controls in a law and order system and they're not going to let you tamper with that.

The other problem would be the media. All you need is one horror story, one person who walks out of here and does some harm. Even if you could open the hospital that would do it. You'd be the bad guy and the D.C.Commissioners would step in and close you down." He paused for a moment, shook his head and said, "I just don't think it can be done."

9

Planning to unlock the hospital

My first act, as Chief, was to announce that every unit was going to house both sexes. It caused quite a stir throughout the building. The nurses on the female wards were very alarmed, and their patients only slightly less so. Paul Barnes, George Hall, and Helen Shea had their work cut out for them in restoring some degree of equanimity before the big day. On the male side the news was received more favorably and preening became the order of the day. Men who had shaved irregularly, as an afterthought with heavy staff prompting, were converted to daily use of the razor, and after-shave lotion came into vogue. Passes for trips to the barbershop were requested even without staff reminders.

It was as if the whole place were awakening to a new day. Men and women who had been content to lounge in pajamas for weeks at a time were dressing up for breakfast and staying that way until bedtime. Patients called home to upgrade their wardrobes and as a result family members arrived at all hours of the day with fresh supplies. We already had daily visiting hours but we now adopted anytime visiting, as long as it didn't interfere with events in the treatment program.

By D-Day everyone in the building was in street clothes and it had a powerful impact on the staff. Patients were showing a new respect for themselves and for one another, and the nurses decided that they too would don street clothing and shed their former authoritarian attire.

We had become a building of equals to the significant benefit of both patients and staff. Those much feared sexual transgressions by the men never occurred, not even the slightest one. Instead they abandoned the use of obscene language and gave up barracks talk both in the corridors and their own bedrooms. The women suddenly displayed a new sexual decorum themselves. It was now safe for any man to encounter them on the wards without the danger of sexual solicitation. We were beginning to look like a hospital that could safely open its doors. The transition from wards segregated by sex to mixed was like going from a primitive society to one more civilized, from crude to polite. We had underestimated the powerful therapeutic effect men and women would have on each other. There was another reason why the move went so smoothly and that was because our wards were now less crowded. Even while we were preparing to integrate the sexes we were reaping the benefits of a new admissions policy that Jim Foy had established almost casually in one of his last staff meetings.

The topic on that occasion had been the lengthy delay between the time patients arrived in the main emergency room and their admission to psychiatry. Our poor patients had to survive a waiting period of up to 12 hours in one of the most chaotic environments in the city. They were competing for attention with the victims of gunshot wounds and stabbing whose stretchers were sometimes lined up in gridlock. Psychiatric patients usually came with a best friend who was in fact their most important link to reality. By the time of admission many of these companions had fallen by the wayside.

One of the classic stories of D.C. General Hospital was the patient whose chart was inscribed with the words: "Coma of Unknown Origin. Arrived in coma with a friend, and the friend left." Life was like that in the big city hospital. We often started treatment from the bottom of a deep hole facing a perilous ascent without much help from the outside.

We took that for granted, but fortunately Jim Foy did not. Someone asked him why it was that our patients had to be seen in the main emergency room before admission. He looked puzzled for a moment as though he had just been asked why the hospital was located on 19th Street Southeast where it had always been. He began his reply with, "Well, it's an old medical tradition. You want to evaluate patients carefully before you bring them into the hospital and the ER is the best place to do it, quickly if it has to be, and thoroughly. Now in our case it's important to be sure there isn't some terrible physical condition, like a brain tumor or a head injury, before people get admitted to psychiatry and so the medical staff in the ER has to look them over first."

He paused here and I could see that the wheels were turning over in his mind. They were turning over in my mind too, and in the minds of all the other MD's in the room. Jim continued: "You know for most of the services they call one of their doctors right away to come over and decide about admission. For our patients the ER staff does the medical screening and then they send them over here. John Schultz and Mary MacIndoo always thought this system worked to our advantage, and all of us did back then. But times have changed. The more I think about it, they're really sort of questioning our medical judgment."

Dr.Luke Grande, our newest staff member, was first to speak for the collective mind, and almost jumped out of his chair in anger. "It's an insult, we're doctors too. Why can't we do our own screenings? Patients who arrive over there for psychiatric help should be sent here right away." The sentiment was unanimous.

"I'll call the Medical Director and get his O.K.", said Jim Foy. "I'm almost certain he'll approve. He's got a big overload problem in the emergency room and this will help reduce the waiting list. We'll set up our own medical admitting office in the basement."

And thus it came about. It was obvious from the start that most of our patients had come through the main emergency room with a companion who now came along to help them find our building. At first this circumstance made little difference in the admissions procedure. Family members and friends were simply pleased at the new ease of access to a hospital.

What was happening was that the resident doctors who met them in our new Admitting Office were operating under their own time constraints, and eager to make a decision about admission as soon as possible. They weren't inclined to bring a third person into the decision-making process, and were routing patients into the hospital based on the degree of overt psychosis evident in the patient. In other words, the residents were doing just what they shouldn't be doing in terms of trying to get through to their patients. Companions were being treated like part of the scenery.

We decided the residents needed some help since they often were dealing with a backup of persons to be seen. Graduate nurses were too busy to leave their wards and social workers were gone by 4:30 pm. There was only one group available to assist with admissions, the good, old reliable nursing assistants.

If we had planned it that way, which we hadn't, things could not have turned out better. At first the nursing assistants stood by and talked with the patient's friend while the resident physician carried out his assessment. With the wealth of information gained in that interval, they quickly became engaged with patients while the doctors were writing their notes. It might be more accurate to say they became involved in a huddle with both patient and companion, in which a degree of animation began to replace flattened affect in someone already assigned to a ward. If there had been any question before this time it now became very clear that our nursing assistants were the best people at getting through with inner warmth in the building. It wasn't long before we changed our admission routine to maximize the interface between our gifted nursing staff and patients. The former became the first in line to meet new arrivals, so their empathic resources could be tapped to get inside these people and assess their needs.

Admission to the hospital became a very personal matter. Patients and companions were registered by an admissions clerk who was himself a good greeter. He would determine if they already knew any member of the nursing staff, or if they could recall someone familiar from a prior hospitalization. They were given the option of seeing such a person or else one of the staff from the ward to which they would be assigned. A new warmth, and sometimes levity, came into being in the admission conference.

It hadn't really occurred to us how often those who brought people to the hospital were also the same ones who had been helping them to maintain a tenuous hold on reality. Illness had eroded these relationships to the point where they were almost moribund. The nursing assistants were breathing new life into patients and new hope and readiness to help into their companions. Some were beginning to recover on our very doorstep.

As they became reanimated, prospective patients were invited to see the ward in which they would stay before signing into the hospital. After such a visit a new option was now made available to many of them. They could remain on that ward or go home with what I called our Gold Bond Guarantee that a bed was being reserved in their name for occupancy at any hour of the day or night. There would be no waiting, no red tape. With that kind of reassurance and encouragement, many elected to return home, and our wards finally acquired some welcome breathing space.

The therapeutic potential of friends and family re-awakened our interest in developing a volunteer service. About a year before we had made our first serious attempt at public outreach without very good results. On that occasion we had been presented with what looked like a great opportunity for a public relations coup. A regional meeting of the American Medical Association was to take place in Washington, D.C. We mounted an exhibit for it touting the advantages of early hospitalization for severe mental illness.

Several hundred physicians viewed the color photographs showing our warm and friendly interior space, and detailing our treatment program. Most were unmoved and their response was at best underwhelming. One internist whom I knew said, "You can't fool us with those pictures. That place is filled with zombies." We were still a leper colony right in the middle of the District in the minds of many.

My wife, who is one of the most enthusiastic volunteers of all time, offered to develop the volunteer service for us. Thanks to the generosity of the local radio stations we soon had announcements about our needs, playing at all hours of the day. Our staff members heard them both while driving in and going home and their morale suddenly became sky-high. Patients heard them on their radios and were delighted. Help was on the way, but the real reason for the boost in everyone's spirits was that we were now being identified as a good place to go to, rather than a lock-up for people who couldn't behave properly in the community.

One of the first groups to respond to my wife's many phone calls was a collection of Georgetown college students who offered to put on a "Hootenanny" for our patients. This was a kind of Country-Western show with colorful costumes, stories, jokes, and guitar music. There were lots of songs with sing-along opportunity. We decided to hold it in our splendid auditorium as an appropriate inaugural for patient use of the facility.

When my wife and I arrived for the evening performance there was already a good scattering of patients who had come down to the first floor auditorium on their own. We spotted a woman seated by herself who was known to the staff as "the great stone face", and we were able to occupy the two seats next to her. Her face was almost immobile as though cast in concrete with a prominent jaw that rarely moved for the purpose of speech. She was a person of great mystery to the staff, as she had disclosed almost nothing about herself during a whole week in the hospital. She had a job but wanted to give it up because she didn't like it, and wished to go to St. Elizabeth's Hospital as a voluntary admission. From her behavior and very few comments, she had not appeared to be psychotic. I introduced my wife to her, and she barely nodded in her direction. I tried to engage her in some conversation regarding the show we were about to see, but without success. She sat silently through the first fifteen minutes of the event and then I became aware that her eyes were moist and she was crying ever so softly. I said to her quietly, "I can see that the show has touched you," and she replied with great feeling, "Yes, they're doing all this for us. They're trying so hard to make us feel good." With that she began to sing and continued to do so with gusto and a bright smile for the rest of the evening. Between songs she confided to me that her feelings had been "frozen" for the past year, and that her son and daughter had moved to another part of the country and remained out of touch. Her loneliness had been unbearable. After the show I escorted her back to the ward and she began a lengthy conversation with her nurse that led ultimately to a reunion with her children. She left us to move to a small town in California, opting for a more appropriate home than St. Elizabeth's that was much closer to her children.

The huge success of the Hootenanny was followed in about a month by an even more uplifting endeavor, an evening visit to all of the wards by the choir of the Georgetown Visitation Convent School for girls, singing Christmas carols by candlelight. For many of our patients it was a once-in-a-life-time kind of experience, arranged for by the President of the Visitation Alumnae, Mrs. Priscilla Ryan.

Our search for volunteers took us to some interesting places one of which I think of to this day. A Baptist Minister, who was already helping out by running errands for patients with his car, asked me if I would want to attend a special meeting of his colleagues to tell them about our program. As I was to learn, the gathering was actually held to allow them to try out some of their material for sermons to be delivered on the following Sunday.

I was looking for the familiar sight of my friend's black sedan as I approached the downtown church where the meeting was to occur. He had really given us a lift with that car, and many of our patients had gotten much more than transportation from their rides with him. Suddenly I saw about thirty black four-door sedans in a Church parking lot, and I knew that I was in the right place. To passersby it was simply a full parking lot. I saw it as a mighty armada of ships of mercy.

The church was large and it had to be because it contained a steep amphitheater around which the ministers were scattered in groups of two or three. One of their number was holding forth with a powerful and moving sermon as I sat down. While they took their turns, I realized what an extraordinary privilege it was for me to be there. At Regis High oratorical skills were prized beyond belief. These men were absolute virtuosos at their craft. Their rhetoric soared and plunged, commanding attention at every moment, and reaching directly into the very soul. The devotion of these gifted preachers to their spiritual cause was powerfully uplifting.

Over the course of the morning I met a good many of the group, and I was impressed by the similarity of their professional goals with my own as a doctor. They listened intently to what I had to say about our hospital, and expressed a genuine appreciation for our efforts, assuring me that we could count on their parishioners for support. On my arrival I had been quite conscious of the fact that I was the only white person in the Church, but as I left I had been made to feel like one of their brothers.

By their very presence our volunteers enhanced the self-respect of patients. Their actions gave living testimony to the valued status of those whom they came to serve. They liked our patients and were not afraid of them, showing them in this way that they needn't be fearful of themselves, and could like whom they were.

We were almost ready to become the first hospital of its kind in this country to open all its doors, but to do so we had to gain the approval of the Chief Judges of the D.C. Superior Court and the U.S. District Court. Over 500 of our admissions each year were faced with a wide variety of criminal charges in court and so we had to ask both judges and prosecutors to make their own decision about the potential danger to society if these people were to be placed in an unlocked hospital.

We already had an unusually good rapport with the prosecutors, many of who were friends of mine from Georgetown Law School days. They knew that our staff shared their concern for the safety of the public and that we were willing to do consultations in jail, if necessary, to become an open hospital.

Getting approval from Chief Judge John L. Smith of the Superior Court would be a harder task. He was not only a strong law and order person, but had recently called us on the carpet for inadequate supervision of one of his court referrals. Still, from courtroom experience, we knew him to be a reasonable man and careful listener. We would have to present a well-reasoned case to win his support.

As it turned out, the statute in the D.C. Code that authorized judges to send people to us for 30-day evaluations actually ordered us to provide psychiatric treatment during that time. We based our plea on this clear mandate. Since we MUST provide treatment, it had to be the most effective kind possible and we had already concluded, on solid clinical evidence, that this required an unlocked setting. Judge Smith had done his own homework and he was well prepared with questions regarding the clinical evidence. For about half an hour he gave us a masterful lesson in the art of judicial inquiry. He seemed to know just what to ask about every aspect of our operation and we found ourselves telling him everything there was to say, including some things we hadn't intended to say. Without even demanding it he was getting the whole truth and nothing but the truth. He finally settled back in his chair and said, "All right I think I've got the whole picture," whereupon he took a deep breath and exhaled slowly.

"I'll be honest about it," he said, "I'm a little scared about the idea of opening your doors. Over the years we've had a number of incidents of people coming out of that place and doing some harm. I'm still thinking about the drug addict I put in your custody, and a week later he was out on the street pushing dope."

Admitting our error on that one, we informed the judge of our decision to keep addicts referred from court on our locked alcoholic detoxification unit for 30 days before their return to court. His Honor nodded approvingly and continued, "Well, I've checked with the other judges to see if they've had any problems with D.C. General lately, and I've gotten some good reports. They're seeing a difference in attitude now when people come back from the hospital. I'm impressed by what you've told me this morning about your new programs, and I don't want to stand in the way of progress. As far as I'm concerned you can unlock the hospital, but if there's any trouble you'll have to be ready to close it back up again."

Encouraged by our meeting with Judge Smith, we arranged for one with Chief Judge Matthew McGuire of the Federal District Court. Our staff was extremely pessimistic about the prospects for a successful outcome to that conference, and I knew the reason why. All of us had had to testify in the Federal District Courthouse on at least a few occasions, and it was a daunting experience. The building itself is a massive structure of concrete and granite occupying a whole square block of the District of Columbia at the foot of Capitol Hill. Unlike the Superior Court that was a veritable beehive of people, its vaulted corridors were hushed so that you could hear your footsteps on the marble floors. The few people present were usually in pairs and engaged in very quiet and serious conversation. Expert witnesses were ushered into small rooms where they smoked, talked minimally and nervously, and waited endlessly, glancing at their watches every five minutes.

Then came the great moment when a court official appeared at the door to call your name and escort you down the hall and through the double doors into the arena of justice. In a well-publicized case there might be 50-100 spectators seated on the benches that occupied the back half of a spacious paneled courtroom. The front half was dominated by a massive wooden altar of justice, which had boxes for a witness, court clerk and stenographer at the base and an elevated platform to house the black-robed judge and his desk. Two large tables, well stacked with books and documents were at the disposal of the defense and prosecution teams in the well before the altar of justice. The judge's weighty presence was a highly visible centerpiece to the whole dramatic scene.

As any witness would soon learn, a Federal District Judge is a person of awesome power when on the bench. He is the final arbiter of everything that transpires in the trial, including the quality, length and intelligibility of your testimony. He is the overseer of courtroom etiquette: "Now doctor you'll have to speak more loudly so the jury can hear". "Just answer the attorney's question, and don't go beyond it". "Don't argue with the prosecutor."

It takes time and experience to learn the mores of courtroom testimony. Until one does you have to expect to deal with the barbs of an exasperated judge who already had his hands full trying to quiet the acrimony between the contesting lawyers. The testifying psychiatrist is likely to take some hits from all sides but the grilling by the black-robed figure who sits on high is often the most well remembered trauma. All of our doctors had been through this mill, leading them to expect a hard time from the Chief Judge. On the day of the meeting at least three of them came by my office to offer their condolences in advance. It was as if I were going to face the Wizard of Oz with a petition of dubious merit.

Judge McGuire proved to be rather different from the ogre of our fantasy. He began the conference by telling me about a conversation that he had had in the week before with Professor Ken Pye of the Georgetown University Law School. Prof. Pye had developed a unique legal internship program at Georgetown, and his trainees were acquiring a very favorable reputation in the U.S. District Court. The Judge had learned that I was giving them some seminars with the professor on Durham Rule psychiatric testimony and he wanted to hear all about what we were doing.

After a lengthy discussion of this topic he spoke of his fondness for the Law School and his own experiences in teaching there. We talked about some of the courses I had taken there including especially Edward Bennett Williams' course in criminal law.

A lot of time had gone by and up to that point there had been no mention of D.C. General by either one of us. The Judge finally broached the subject, saying, "Now about this open hospital, I've already sent a memo to the other judges telling them that you'll be unlocking the wards and the building pretty soon. You have our support. After all, you're one of us. You belong to the legal profession as well as the medical, and we trust your judgment. You can go ahead whenever you're ready, but there's just one thing". And here he touched on the theme of every Chief Psychiatrist's nightmares. "As long as there are no notorious incidents." The Wizard of Oz had spoken and it turned out he was just a friendly man from Kansas.

We were on the brink of unlocking every door in our building but a few anxious moments remained. We were very mindful of the fact that the judges' unanimous verdict in our favor had the caveat about notorious incidents. On the Friday afternoon before Monday's scheduled opening the tranquility of the first floor was shattered by a series of piercing screams that emanated from the admitting office on the level below. The reverberations shook the Chief Psychiatrist and Nursing Supervisor from their office redoubts in a race to the elevator.

As we headed towards the four-alarm commotion in the basement the words "notorious incident" were running through my mind. "Are we really ready for Monday?" I asked Helen Shea.

Her reply was, "I'm wondering about that, too, but we've come too far to turn back. Don't worry we'll be all right. As for the man screaming in the admitting office, I can tell you all about him because I was there when he came in and we have a lot of background history." Her account follows in summary fashion.

The patient was a 23-year-old man, brought in by two D.C. police-men who had seen him wandering on a downtown street making strange noises. On arrival he was somewhat incoherent, his unkempt hair and attire in equal disarray. He had a wild look in his eyes and was hearing "voices" that seemed to be the source of an explosive degree of inner turmoil. The resident doctor could make no sense out of what he was saying, and told him that this was so. He suggested that it must be because the patient himself was experiencing so much confusion in his own mind. The latter agreed quite readily with this, and seemed to be relieved when it was recommended that he stay in the hospital to get some help with his confusion. The resident was able to reach an uncle by telephone and soon learned the explanation for a series of incoherent remarks that the patient had been making about a roommate.

It seems that his nephew had been a "loner", a very shy man with few friends, perhaps indeed only one, the man with whom he had shared his apartment for the past two years. Together, they had developed a small electronics business, the patient being the "genius in the back room" and his roommate, the garrulous salesman and "public contacts man." They had gone to the same college, but barely knew each other there, their friendship having started when his roommate arrived in Washington without a place to live. The uncle referred to the latter as a scoundrel, who "used people for all they were worth," and only recently had informed his nephew of his intention to move to California. The uncle surmised that the partner might be one jump ahead of the sheriff because of some of his questionable business practices, but allowed that it was even more likely that he was having girlfriend trouble because he was one of the most notorious womanizers in Washington. In this regard, he chuckled and said that he didn't dare repeat some of the sto-ries that his nephew had told him. The uncle guessed that his nephew had lived vicariously through the partner since he had no social life of his own with women. His main life interest had been his work to which he had devoted twelve to fourteen hours a day.

With this information, the resident tried to talk with the patient, Mr. Y, about the impact of the imminent departure of such an important person in his life, but to no avail. Efforts to approach the subject seemed only to generate more confusion in the patient. The doctor accordingly shifted to the topic of work, and found him to be somewhat enthusiastic about the prospect that he might use some of his skills in a regular hospital job, in our "work therapy" program. They also discussed the matter of a ward government assignment, and here the patient had selected the clean-up committee, hoping to get a chance to operate the giant buffer that he had seen used in the admitting room. Pleased with the degree of contact he had been able to establish, the resident had announced that he would see him on the next day. He added that Mr. Y could go up to the ward with a nursing assistant; whereupon the patient began to emit a series of loud bellowing noises that literally shook our building. His blasts were in the form of the sounds of "OH" and "OW"—almost inhuman in quality, yet faintly suggestive of the expression of a gigantic degree of surprise and pain.

By the time we got to the admitting office, the resident had begun to make some headway in learning about the eerie noises that were now issuing forth from Mr. Y at more protracted intervals. The resident introduced us, told us that his patient was very confused, and that it might have something to do with the departure of his roommate. He provided a verbatim report of the uncle's comments, but noted that now Mr. Y had a new problem. "He says that there is a psychiatrist inside of him who is carrying out a physical examination." "Yes," the patient said, "He just came in my ear. He says 'you need to be reamed out in here. I'm going to send for a roto rooter. Now he's down in my stomach". He's saying "It's empty in here and it's dark." Suddenly, in a loud voice, the patient shouted "Hello-oo-o up there. I almost got lost. I'm in the gallbladder now. Wow, there sure is a lot of gall in here."

At that point, the resident's eyes lit up signaling his own internal illumination, and he said, "Mr. Y, the psychiatrist must be confused. It sounds like he thinks he's in your roommate's gallbladder. He has more gall than anybody in Washington from what your uncle told me."

Looking first stunned and then tearful, the patient responded slowly and thoughtfully, "He has all the gall and I have none. What am I going to do. It's just too much for me to think about. When can I go to work on the other side of the hospital?"

"You'll have to be able to keep from yelling so loudly," Helen Shea observed gently.

"You're right, I was roaring. I lost control. I must have been crazy. I've been afraid of going crazy. So many weird things happening in my life. The doctor was causing me a lot of pain poking around in there. Or was that real? I've got to get some things figured out. I need to be here, but I don't want to just sit around."

He was speaking now in well-modulated and friendly tones, without the wild-eyed look or tormented blasts. Turning to the resident, he asked quite calmly, "Can we talk some more today?" To which the latter replied, "Of course. We have a lot to talk about. I'll see you on the unit in a half-hour." And the room heaved a sigh of relief.

I thought about Mr. Y's own observation that he had been "roaring" and had lost control. His uncle's comment that he had been living vicariously through his roommate was in the right direction, but inadequate to convey the deep merger by which this man had actually become a component of his make-up. And so the partner's decision to leave had caused a splintering of the patient's psychic structure, which released some of those primitive, destructive, drive energies that characterize the human beast in his untamed state. The patient had, indeed, been roaring, like a lion about to pounce on his prey perhaps, or an inferno blazing out of control. His rage had become diffuse. If it had had even some initial focus towards his roommate, much of it had been turned back on himself, producing depression and depersonalization, and finally almost total withdrawal from the real world.

Once his rage had been internalized, it was no longer a menacing force directed towards his roommate and the rest of the world. It had spared his own life, too, but had almost destroyed him as a person. His most immediate need was to feel like a person again, and the resident doctor, by his gentle efforts to make contact, his ability to convey some understanding of the patient's own inner experience, and his ready acceptance and support of the latter's strengths had already facilitated the restoration of personhood. But then came the doctor's abrupt announcement of their parting, like a thunder-clap in the patient's stormy interior to which he responded with a psychotic solution to the danger of abandonment. He swallowed a psychiatrist. (Here we can see how this delusion tended to achieve the disguised fulfillment of a number of important wishes, much in the manner of the 'normal' dreaming process.) His roommate was deserting him. He had found a potential replacement, who now also threatened to leave. And so he took the new power-figure inside to guard against the loss, and work over the pain that the resident was causing.

After about a week in the hospital, Mr. Y was able to confide in his doctor about a worry that had been causing him a great deal of shame. He asked his doctor to look at a small crease in his abdominal wall, just below the navel. The resident reassured him that it was a perfectly normal variation that could be found somewhere in the skin of everyone. Mr. Y then told him that he was so ashamed of it that he hadn't wanted anyone to see it. He was convinced that his body was beginning to undergo a series of changes that would lead him to develop breasts like a woman, and cause his penis to be replaced with a woman's genital.

The delusion that a man's body is undergoing a sexual transformation is a psychiatric classic, often found in paranoid schizophrenia. Freud wrote about it in the case of Schreber, a distinguished judge, who felt that God was working such a change in his body for cosmic purposes. Freud cited this delusion in support of his belief that sexual conflicts were at the root of that illness. Most analysts would now regard it as simply part of an elaborate defense against a biologically determined upsurge of destructive drive energies.

The resident doctor had been able to establish a substantial degree of human contact with him by the simple and direct communication, "You are confused." Why was this so effective? For one thing, the patient was struggling with a rapid proliferation of delusional ideas and auditory hallucinations in a frantic effort to cope with his own fragmentation and rage. And so his difficulty in sorting out what was real from what was not had produced a profound confusion that was, in fact, what was uppermost in his mind. His confusion was that aspect of the real world in which he had the greatest emotional investment. His doctor, like the mother of a one-year-old, had been able to recognize his confused state and express it verbally for him without even having had to be told about it in words. And finally, the resident had noticed his own mental stumbling, which had arisen as a direct projection from his patient, so that they had already begun to have the kind of intimate bond that comes from a sharing of parts of each other.

Another kind of mental bond came into play when the doctor's intuition allowed him to see that he was fanning the fires by his questions about the roommate. His easy shift to the topic of work fostered a rapprochement that permitted him to share with enthusiasm in the ensuing discussion about job opportunities in the hospital. Mr. Y did get to push the big buffer, and his doctors' steady approval helped him to convert its masculinizing currents into a durable part of his self-esteem. Mr. Y also opted to join the greeting committee of his ward. He told his doctor that this might help him to be less shy, and that he was an expert in the matter of arriving at the hospital in a state of utter confusion.

Mr. Y's case illustrates the usefulness of our work therapy program, which was one of the key reasons for our rapid arrival on the brink of becoming an open hospital. It had begun a few years earlier under the guidance of Ms. Frances Mason who nurtured it carefully in its first years, and had it in a thriving condition by the time of Mr. Y's arrival. Patients were offered the chance to work as volunteers in a variety of jobs in the other divisions of the D.C. General as well as in our own building.

At the outset only a few were given this opportunity, usually people who had been there some time and lived on the open ward. But in the past year the staff had begun to make many more referrals, some even on the first or second hospital day as in the case of Mr. Y. There were now as many as forty patients coming and going from the locked wards each day. In other words we were already 20% open.

Frances Mason had gotten to know every supervisor throughout the hospital, and was very familiar with their personal strengths and weaknesses. She was adept at matching patients with the right supervisors and work situations. For Mr. Y she chose the Administrator's Office because it had a congenial staff who could make him feel at home, and some projects that would challenge his problem-solving skills. Mirabile dictu, this man emerged from the total mental chaos, and physical disarray of Friday to find the solution to a baffling inventory dilemma on the following Wednesday.

The administrator's office had been struggling for ten years to find a way to keep tabs on the hospital's supply of sheets and towels. In just five days Mr. Y's skill at writing programs for computers produced a foolproof system. His rapid-fire mind worked somewhat like the computerized gadgets he had been called on to repair in his shop. When he left the hospital four weeks later, he was offered a job in the Administrator's Office that he declined, to return to his beloved electronics business.

Mr. Y was not the only graduate of the work therapy program to receive a job offer from the hospital, there were many others. The man he had seen pushing a buffer in our entrance hall on his first day became a valued member of the housekeeping staff in the surgical division. It was always a pleasure to run into him over there. He operated his machine with such an evident contentment in his work, always smiling and singing songs to himself.

How important is daily work to the maintenance of a sound mind? "Very," was the answer we received over and over again. Our work therapy program was a powerful lever that could lift people out of the depths of depression and regression, and back into active participation in the real world. The daily work efforts of forty people had also lifted a hospital and all its patients to the brink of a whole new way of life.

10

The miracle of D.C. General

The doors opened wide on that fateful Monday to the accompaniment of much staff trepidation. Patients were free now to wander off the wards for a breath of fresh air, or take the pedestrian tunnel to the main hospital without awaiting the assistance of someone with a key. They could slip out the back door for a stroll down to the Anacostia River or walk freely onto the nursing station to chat with its occupants. The ward offices were no longer locked and even those in "seclusion" rooms could emerge at will. We had declared ourselves and our patients to be on equal footing with everyone else in the D.C. General Hospital.

And yet we were still a big city hospital faced with the admission of 3,000 patients per year, most of whom were acutely psychotic. Police cars would still roll in with outraged White House cases, and teams of policemen would still grapple with patients on our doorstep. There would be other Mr. Y's plucked from the city's streets, and other Eddies arriving with tearful mothers at home. Would it work to be so open?

Helen Shea was busy receiving bulletins in the coffee room and I decided to hit the wards. Stepping off the elevator on the third floor I was greeted with a most unusual sight. There was Dr. Paul Barnes, Chief Medical Officer of Unit Three, seated on a straight-backed chair staring at the open door to his domain. "Good morning, Paul," I said, "Are we going to watch the Redskins practice at noon today?" (Their practice field was right next door to our building in that era and Paul and I were frequent spectators.)

"Don't make jokes Jim", he replied. "This is serious business. We don't know what's going to happen today and I'm not taking any chances.

We've got a couple of people who might just decide to take off and I'm going to be here to greet them if they do."

I commiserated with Paul and told him I was as anxious as he, and trying to walk mine off by touring the building.

"Well," he said, "You'll see George Hall out on his chair on the fourth floor, but I don't know what you'll find on the fifth. Luke Grande is probably on the inside rapping with his patients. I can hear him now. 'Listen if you want to leave, here is your chance, but don't!…'"

Noon came and no one had tried to leave, and there certainly had been no notorious incidents. Paul and I met for lunch at our accustomed time and place to watch our favorite team.

By unlocking the units, we had also embarked on a closer and more caring relationship with our patients. There was now a greater intimacy with them. They could walk along with staff members going to the sandwich shop in the main hospital, or join the rest of the Redskins fans on the sidelines. Experiences at home could be shared with staff right after they happened. We had given our patients a tremendous vote of confidence in their ability to control their behavior. They, in turn, boosted our conviction that we could be of help to almost any kind of patient.

Four weeks after the opening, I had an urgent request for some back-up help from a nearby psychiatric hospital that taught me even more about the character of our staff. The call came around nine at night. It was from Dr. Joe Costa who was on the psych ward at Fairfax Hospital in Northern Virginia, and in the midst of a turbulent situation. He had a man there who was suicidal but had reached an impasse with the staff and wanted to sign out. His family was present and he was willing to go to another hospital with them but as Joe put it, "There's just too much bad chemistry on both sides for him to stay here. Can you take him?"

Joe was a good clinician, conscientious physician and also a friend. He had been in charge of the addiction program at D.C. General before his entry into full-time private practice two years before. My first reaction to his call went unspoken, but I was thinking to myself, "Whoa! It's nine o'clock. We have a shift change due at eleven. You have him on a locked ward where at least he could stay overnight. Why should we take over your suicide watch, and on an open ward at that?" Friendship won out. I still thought it highly unlikely that we would accept this patient for the reasons just stated, but I also saw Joe's problem: Suicidal patient on a ward where he hates the staff. That's a serious business.

I told him that I didn't think we'd be able to take his patient but that I would call the admitting ward at D.C. General to see what things were like there. I planned to make it clear to their staff that I was not asking them to admit this patient and just wanted to see if they could help in the event of an absolute emergency. I was frankly expecting a rejection.

Mr. Harper, a veteran nursing assistant, took the call and responded with a quick assessment of the patient. "Doc, that man is really in trouble. He wants to kill himself and he doesn't trust the people who are taking care of him. He needs to come in here tonight. Tell Dr. Costa to send him over, we have some bed space. We'll watch him closely and we won't let his family go 'til we know he's O.K. here." I wished that I could have reacted like Mr. Harper, but then I asked myself did I know of any other hospital that would have relieved one of their neighbors of that kind of responsibility at eleven at night. The answer was no.

The Chief Psychiatrist had been handed an object lesson in charity by a civil servant who loved his work and loved his patients. It was a reminder that we are all servants, and caring is the principal coin of our realm. Over the months ahead I had occasion to think of that evening many times as D.C. General began to receive pleas for assistance with difficult patients from the psych wards at Sibley, and the George Washington and Howard University hospitals. They were locked and we were open, but when they felt under pressure to transfer a patient they knew they could count on us to be a willing recipient.

The improved morale of patients and staff gave rise to some interesting projects. It wasn't long after the integration of the sexes that the home-making instincts of the women came to life, and they began to plan the redecoration of our premises. They wanted to make drapes to hide the heavy steel security screens in the building, and beyond that they hoped to acquire floor and table lamps to brighten the dayrooms. Both of these tasks would take money and there was very little available in our tiny volunteer fund. We needed a source of revenue.

Starbucks wasn't the first organization to find that there was a huge profit margin in selling cups of coffee. Our patients at D.C. General discovered this secret 20 years before them. The proposal to start a patient-run coffee service emanated from one of the ward meetings and quickly gained the support of the other units. It started out as a modest endeavor focused on visitors who might pass through our lobby in midday. The number of volunteers available to run the project was enormous so that it soon became possible for the vendors to circulate through all the wards, and the hours were extended from 7:00 AM to 6:00 PM. The availability of coffee at such an early hour of the day captured the incoming staff market. They gladly turned over the preparation chores to the service, which then took over the operation of our coffee room. Patients and staff began to have coffee together and got to know each other much better. The modest coffee proposal had had a powerful unifying effect for both staff and patients who now moved about the building more freely to visit friends from other units. It proved to be a marvelous source of dollars, but better yet it was a priceless asset for meeting our patients' greatest need, good human contact with one another.

The drapery project rolled into high gear with the influx of coffee money, and the sewing machines were soon whirring night and day, on the wards and in the Occupational Therapy Department. Patient seamstresses eventually disguised every security screen in the building with yards of cloth, and at no expense to the District government. New lamps began to appear in the dayrooms—one at a time, since they were being paid for in cash from the coffee tills. And then we had a stroke of luck in the form of a major contribution from our next-door neighbor, the D.C. Jail.

We learned that there was a paint crew composed of inmates who were available to work on properties owned by the District of Columbia. Our request for a repainting of the entire building was granted and the results were spectacular. Dr. Bernie Levy, Chief Psychologist, had a gifted color sense and personally supervised the preparation of every gallon of paint applied to the walls. He insisted that each unit be done in its own distinctive pastel color and he added special pigments to every can of paint. Doors were finished in a contrasting darker hue. To complete the whole project, Bernie teamed up with Ms. Elinor Ullman, one of the pioneers of art therapy, to select appropriate works of art for display about the building.

It was fascinating to see how the crew of prisoners worked themselves into the therapeutic ambience of our hospital. They befriended patients on all the wards, made suggestions at ward meetings and attended AA sessions whenever possible. By the end of their stay they left with heads held high, proud of their work and strengthened by their good experiences with our patients.

It was not long afterward that I had a great awakening. One of the Chief Psychiatrist's duties under the D.C. Code had been to sign a daily form for each patient who had been subjected to any kind of physical restraint, attesting to his knowledge that restraints had been used. When I joined the staff there might have been as many as ten or twelve of these; the number gradually declined over the years to one or two by the time we integrated the sexes.

One morning I glanced at my desktop for the forms and an alarm bell went off. I hadn't signed one of these documents in over two weeks. There was a moment of bureaucratic panic as I weighed the impact of my lapse on the Nursing Administrator's Office, and I called Helen Shea to see how we could make amends to her Supervisor. Her response was to laugh at my worry and then she said, "There hasn't been anyone in restraints for the past couple of weeks. I forgot to tell you. When you decided to open the hospital one of the first questions in our nursing meeting was, 'What do we do if someone in restraints wants to leave?' We got to thinking about how and why people are put in restraints over the next few weeks and the nursing assistants really led the way in these discussions. They kept making the point that if you have to put someone down it means you haven't made contact with them, and that's what their job is all about, to get through to people. They finally reached the conclusion that it represents a failure on their part if a person is put in restraints, and since then no one has been in restraints. I've got my fingers crossed." In fact there was no one in restraints for the remainder of our life as an open hospital.

After the nursing assistants had shown us the way on the matter of restraints they turned their attention to another topic that the rest of us had not yet begun to think about. The doors were now open on the nursing stations, but they questioned the need for the thick glass panels that still surrounded the enclosures. "Why do we have those barriers separating us from the patients?" they asked with perfect logic. I had no answer for that, but wasn't in any hurry to think about such a monumental structural change. It wasn't too long before Helen Shea approached me with a request from her nursing staff to have the panels removed. Convinced by then that it was a good idea, I forwarded a requisition to the Administrator's Office. It came back with a strange note attached: "We can't do this now because it would cost too much. Besides we talked with Dr. Schultz and he said, 'Don't do it unless you check with me first." The old fox was back in our territory and I wasn't sure why.

Meanwhile I was noticing less and less people with overt schizophrenia on rounds through the hospital. My way of keeping in touch with the clinical performance of the wards had always been to look for patients with visible schizophrenia and ask the staff about them. Their spontaneous utterances would usually help them to develop a plan for getting through. A good example of one of these mini-conferences came on a day when there were no schizophrenics to be seen. There was an air of tension on a nursing station that seemed a bit odd because the ward itself appeared to be in good shape. "Are you having trouble with someone here?" I asked, and the nurse and her two assistants all began to answer at once. It seems that a man charged with a white-collar crime had been sent in for a court evaluation with a number of restrictions demanded by the U.S. Attorney's Office. He was to remain on the ward itself for 30 days, and visitation was strictly limited to his wife and family. There was a suspicion that he might have some connections with drug dealers although his court charges were not drug-related. To put it mildly the patient was enraged with his caretakers for a set of rules and regulations that were totally at odds with his free-spirited style of life. He was going eyeball-to-eyeball with staff, and withering them with looks that could kill. Worse yet he had engaged in bold confrontations with each of them in which he announced his intention to "take out a contract" on their lives. His explosive inner rage had caused both patients and staff to withdraw from him in fear.

After airing their many grievances one of the nursing assistants asked a very pertinent question: "Why would someone go around telling people over and over again that he wanted to have them killed? He must be very scared himself and he's trying to tell us how powerful he is. He's trying to convince himself that he's strong because he feels so weak and in danger."

The comment seemed to open up a whole new perspective on the patient for his colleagues. The other nursing assistant added: "Everybody up here is so afraid of him that they withdraw and don't want to have anything to do with him. So he really is all alone and abandoned on the ward. He desperately needs some friends but he's afraid of everybody. We've got to try to find some way to show him we're on his side. I think I'll ask him if he needs anything from the canteen today."

"That's a good idea," said his colleague, "He's always looking for a newspaper to read in the morning. I'll start bringing in the Washington Post."

"What he really needs," said the nurse, "is to feel more important. He's smart and he was in charge of a big office before he came in here. He'd be a good person to have as Ward Chairman if only he'd start talking to other people. I think I'll try to talk with him about that."

Each set out to help in his own way, and in two days they reported a remarkable turn-around in which they were hearing all about the patient's family and lifetime in business. Gone were the threats against staff. He started to work on some plans for the ward that led him to become one of the finest ward chairpersons in our history.

I can offer a brief follow-up on this patient because I met him about three months later in jail while doing an evaluation on another inmate.

I was seated alone at a table in the big open rotunda, awaiting the arrival of the examinee when I saw our former patient approaching rapidly with a big smile on his face.

"Dr. Ryan, I'm so glad to see you," he announced as we shook hands. His warmth was clearly genuine and touching. "I'm working in the front office now so I'm free to move around a little. I heard you were coming here two days ago (he knew just about everything that was going on in the building), and I felt I just had to see you. That experience I had at D.C. General was like nothing that's ever happened in my life before. I really felt I was doing something worthwhile and I had the respect of everyone. It was like waking up from a bad nightmare. I had been doing drugs—all kinds, and I had almost destroyed my family and myself. I deserve to be in here just for that but I was also cutting corners with the law on the company books to get money for my habit. I've been going to the NA (narcotics anonymous) meetings here and I'll be even more active with them when I get out. I'm a new person now and I just wanted to thank you and thank the staff at D.C. General. They're wonderful people."

We had been getting some good results with our over 400 court admissions during the year. Some were able to change from a life pattern of frequent troubles with the law, and jail sentences, to a readiness to enter the hospital for brief stays in times of inner distress. Out of 454 referrals, only four had failed to return to court on their appointed trial date. All of these were drifters who had had transient breakdowns on their way through Washington to various southern destinations. The Prosecutor's Office thanked us for helping them to resume their journey and wished them bon voyage.

We were enjoying even greater success with the rest of our admissions. The commitment rate to St. Elizabeth's had dropped from 70% to a virtual zero, save for a few people of advanced age who needed to live in the nursing facility there. We actually had reached the point where I now saw almost no one with overt schizophrenia on my walks through the building. At one of our staff meetings a request from patients to hold a weekly social event for all of the wards came up for consideration. Needless to say we were thrilled by their initiative, and three possible locations for the event were discussed: the doctor's library, our auditorium and the front entrance lobby. After some deliberation, I said "Wait a minute, I think I've got a better idea. The Mental Health Commission Hearing Room is the largest one we have, and of course it has that beautiful paneling and wall to wall carpeting. We could take out the forty chairs, keep the two long tables, and put in a bookcase or two and some comfortable chairs. We'll call it The Patients Lounge. It was not only my best suggestion, but easily the most gratifying.

As word of our unlocking drifted north teams of mental health professionals visited us from two well-known big city hospitals, Philadelphia General and Bellevue in New York. The group from Philadelphia came first, towards the end of our first open year. There were three psychiatrists, a psychologist and a social worker. The site visit was planned as a one-day event.

We began the meeting with a couple of rounds of coffee and donuts from our coffee service (at no charge!). The group listened with great interest to the story of how this cohort of patients had funded our remodeling. We carefully explained that our admissions pool was much the same as theirs, i.e. with 70% being in acutely psychotic states. Following the briefing on all the changes in our program we began a tour of the wards and treatment areas. At each stop the visitors conducted lengthy interviews of several patients, asking us also about their course of treatment. By four in the afternoon we stopped to discuss their observations and questions. They began by stressing how different our hospital was from their own. The wards here were "beautiful", "immaculate", "uncrowded." Patients were all involved in purposeful behaviors, coming and going from the building on a variety of tasks, and frequently engaged in friendly discussions with staff. The latter were perceived as "very alert, eager to help, and enjoying their work." Finally one of their number broached the question that clearly was on the minds of all. "How is it that you have no schizophrenic patients here? Obviously your laws must be much different from ours. Perhaps you're able to send them directly from your emergency room over to St. Elizabeth's or else you just don't have to admit them."

We had to go back over the initial briefing with more explicit details. We told them that we still had some patients who arrived under police escort, and yet we used no restraints. A staff member would sit up with such a patient and work at the task of getting through with inner warmth until they could reach a warming point even if only on a trivial matter. We reviewed with them how we had learned to share warmth with angry White House cases by simply meeting their need for cigarettes, or with mute catatonics by acknowledging their muteness and accepting it as a given. We told them about the lid man and the drugstore waitress. And finally we explained how we had become convinced that schizophrenic withdrawal was really the result of an excess of destructive drive energies, and was a protective mechanism for preventing harm to others. To overcome this withdrawal it was necessary to help patients to reestablish their capacity to share warmth with other human beings, since we had also found that shared warmth was an antidote for rage, and destructive drive energies. Our uncrowded wards resulted from the fact that staff members could often make sufficient contact in admission interviews to help restore a relationship with a companion who then provided ongoing contact that kept the patient out of the hospital.

Our colleagues listened with interest but found it hard to believe that the people we admitted could recover their sanity on the very first hospital day, and maintain it thereafter. We suggested that the original experience of shared warmth with a staff member operated as a first dose of the antidote for the destructive drives. It was therapeutic in itself, but also prepared the way for further dosage with the same medicine from other staff members and even more importantly from other patients. The visitors left with some new ideas but not much hope that they could duplicate our program in the Philadelphia General Hospital. As they said, "We just aren't ready for this and we're not sure if the City Fathers will ever be ready."

A little over one month later a similar contingent of staff members arrived from Bellevue for their inspection of the program. The format was the same although the New Yorkers were more aggressive and probing with their questions and interviewed an even greater number of patients on the wards. In the discussion period at the end of the day, they used almost exactly the same laudatory language to describe what they had seen and again after a polite interval one of the group asked why we had no schizophrenic patients. "Yes," said the rest, "That's the greatest difference between our hospitals, you have no schizophrenic patients and we have nothing but schizophrenic patients." We reminded them that 70% of our patients arrived under the same conditions and in the same mental state as theirs and repeated our explanation for their rapid recovery.

The New Yorkers were unconvinced. After insisting that we must be operating under a different kind of commitment law, they proceeded to outline a number of different ways in which we could be evading the admission of schizophrenics. As we discussed these one-by-one, they began to get a little angry and one even implied that we were not telling the truth. After that things settled down and they described the absolutely chaotic state of their own hospital and the unbearable conditions under which they had been working. As the group exited some of them were waiting for a taxi on our front portico and I could hear their conversation in my office that was immediately adjacent to where they were standing. "There's got to be some way that they're keeping the schizophrenics out. Dr. Ryan just wasn't telling us how they do it." The others echoed the speaker's remarks and off they went in disbelief.

At our staff meeting on the following Monday, I related this anecdote to the great amusement of one and all. Paul Barnes said, "But you know I can understand why they didn't believe you. A year ago there were a bunch of schizophrenics on my ward and now there are none. I still find it very hard to believe what's happened. It's a miracle, that's all. It's just a miracle."

Maybe it was, and maybe it wasn't a miracle. It certainly was an extraordinary human happening and it lasted over a year and a half. When Dr. Jack Ewalt declared that it would be impossible for us to open our doors one of his reasons was our shortage of "qualified" nursing personnel. By any rational standard his appraisal was right. After all, there was only one nurse and two nursing assistants for every forty patients, all of who were acutely disturbed. None of the nurses and their assistants had college degrees and some lacked high school diplomas.

Our own prejudiced misunderstanding of schizophrenics had blinded us to the most powerful therapeutic resource of all, the patients themselves. We started to become aware of their potential as therapists for one another in the ward meetings. It wasn't long in any such gathering before someone would stand up and begin to talk about abusive treatment by "hidden enemies". The other patients would listen attentively even to comments that bordered on the absurd. Many were still dealing with the same kind of delusions although beginning to ask themselves from time to time "if these could be caused by my imagination." They would try to reason with the speaker, try to raise some doubts about what he or she was saying. At the same time they were strengthening their own hold on reality. Eventually the meeting would produce a clear consensus about the flaws in the speaker's thinking. He or she might not be convinced but the meeting could then get on to the real, day-to-day, ward problems that had to be solved. At least the speaker was left with some new perspectives to think about.

The helpful exchanges didn't end with the meeting. People who revealed their delusions in that open forum would find that other patients later approached them to compare notes about their own struggles with worries about "enemies." And if they were afraid to leave the building for fear of harmful plots against them they would have willing escorts among their peers. Our patients were providing one another with an around the clock supply of shared warmth.

We had discovered that schizophrenia was not a hopeless or incurable disease, and that sanity could be restored by an environment that encouraged the sharing of inner warmth with other human beings. We had also learned that all of us, patients and staff alike, possessed a remarkable healing force that was present in the care and concern part of our human nature. The most notable conclusion of the "miracle" of D.C. General was that all human beings are linked with one another by virtue of their care and concern, and the preservation of this linkage is a necessary condition for their rationality. In other words man is not just a rational animal, but primarily a caring animal whose rationality is dependent on the ability to share inner warmth with one another.

11

Human nature's greatest secret, the power to heal

Freud had struggled in vain to make some sense out of the illness of schizophrenia and the closest he could come to it was in his paper "The Case of Schreber", based on the autobiography of a paranoid schizophrenic. Freud provided a richly detailed analysis of Schreber's latent homosexual problems but failed to see that his illness was actually driven by a profound degree of rage that caused him to dream of the destruction of the world. Even Freud had his blindspots when it came to recognizing the toxic potential of human anger. Fortunately he had the gift of prophecy in addition to his psychological skills and so he urged his followers, like Dr. Grete Bibring, to work at solving the mystery of schizophrenia so that we might one day arrive at a new understanding of human nature.

Schizophrenics have an abnormal nervous system chemistry that gives rise to a volatile surplus of aggressive and destructive drive energies. We had good reason to worry about unprovoked violence on the part of our patients at D.C.General. One of our kindest nurses, Chris Welch, had been attacked from behind by a violent woman, who dragged her to the floor, and pulled out a hank of her hair. Luke Grande had been punched in the eye as he approached a patient to say hello. Mr. Alston and Mr. Jerry were the first line of defense against the explosion of catatonic excitement. And then there was the "lid man" whose inner rage had garbled his speech for twenty-four hours before it finally broke through in the urge to kill his roommates. But we learned so much from the "lid man" and from the "White House cases", who were absolutely seething with rage and ready to boil over at any second. We discovered that a "warming point" was possible with everyone, and that when it occurred there was an instant calming of the turbulent energies of the id. The "warming point" was an unmistakable happening. We could see it, hear it, and feel it. The rounds team could agree unanimously about just when it had occurred. The "warming point" was actually the healing event. It gave us a precise new medical definition for healing. Healing occurs when people are able to get through with their inner personal warmth to others whose inner warmth has been depleted, and who are suffering from a surplus of hateful energies. It consists in a taming of the hateful energies. The id had been considered an unreachable source of relentless sexual and aggressive drives that was buried in an unconscious part of the mind. We had learned that a conscious, loving part of the mind could directly modify the id. What a victory for civilization. A hospital where seventy percent of the admissions were struggling with violent urges had proven to be the perfect laboratory for the study of healing.

When we asked ourselves why a warming point could come about so easily we came face to face with the fact that all human beings have a core element of loving energies. These can connect us directly, one with another, for an exchange of loving energies that brings about a warming point. The passageways for the sharing of caring energies can be accessed quite readily under normal circumstances, but they are almost completely shut down by the deep withdrawal from other people seen in schizophrenia. All that was needed to reopen them was to find some simple interest in the real world that had survived their deep withdrawal, and join our patients there. We had discovered that inner personal warmth, a very familiar part of human nature to almost everyone, was actually the most important part of human nature. Our linkage to one another through the bonding power of inner warmth was the very hallmark of human nature.

The healing power of the warming point was awesome. Murderous urges like those in the Lid Man were brought under immediate control. Catatonic pressures to run amok were cured instantly by exposure to the caring energies of a hospital staff. The existence of the healing power of shared inner warmth was a remarkable finding, but even more unexpected was the fact that this wonderful human asset was present in everyone. When we had first raised the question of unlocking the hospital with our consultant, Dr. Jack Ewalt, he said in no uncertain terms that it couldn't be done because our nursing staff was so small. We had only one nurse, and two nursing assistants for every forty patients, most of who had been admitted in very disturbed, psychotic states. As patients regained their ability to share warmth with staff they were soon able to do the same with one another so that healing was going on around the clock for every patient. It was thus that we learned that all of us, patients and staff alike, could be healers through the sharing of inner warmth. This was our most important discovery about human nature.

The precise definition of healing just mentioned is also based on another aspect of human nature revealed at D.C.General, namely that our loving energies are much stronger than our hateful energies and will usually win out when they are matched in a head to head contest. The findings at D.C.General require a re-working of the traditional definition of man as a rational animal. Man is first and foremost a caring animal whose rationality is dependent on having the ability to share care and concern with one another. When this capacity is lost, as in the deep withdrawal of schizophrenia, reality testing is also lost and rationality goes down the tubes. Descarte's famous proclamation in support of his existence, "I think, therefore I am" also deserves revision. "I care, therefore I am" would come closer to the truth.

The staff at D.C.General were also able to observe that their healing outreach of warmth evoked a response of gratitude in patients, rewarding them with an increase in good feelings about their work. In other words their own supply of loving energies was increased. From this it could be seen that healing was always a two-way street, a very important finding indeed, for all of us to think about. We are free to choose whether we use our healing energies or allow them to remain idle. This choice will determine the course of our lives. It marks the difference between a peaceful, happy and secure life, or one that is contentious, disgruntled and worrisome. When we share our inner warmth with others the quality of our life and theirs is enriched. Healing people who are suffering from an overload of hateful or destructive urges provides a fresh supply of caring energies that move us along a pathway to steady emotional growth over a lifetime.

The healing of schizophrenia at D.C.General also cast some fresh light on the destructive drives themselves. We humans have been highly resistant to learning about our own destructive drives, but much more importantly, we can do something to change them. In one respect, the destructive drives are right out there in the open for all of us to see. They are the principal topic of the news media, often graphically displayed or screamed about in the headlines. In wartime we boast about the power of our weapons to destroy. World War Two set a record for daily human carnage that reached a climax in a nuclear holocaust. We know all about the terrible power of the human destructive drives in war, but we simply don't like to recognize them as a part of our individual nature.

Our aversion to knowing about the destructive drives as they exist in ourselves is the reason why schizophrenics have been burned at the stakes as witches, locked up in jails as criminals, herded like cattle into "warehouses for the mentally ill", or left to fend for themselves on the streets. The deep withdrawal of schizophrenics actually gives silent testimony to their inner concern not to harm others. Even though the destructive drives may remain hidden within ourselves, we learned at D.C.General that they are the primary cause of all anxiety and depression. Often an episode of schizophrenia is preceded by several weeks of severe panic and intractable insomnia. Until the destructive drives become blunted by the deep withdrawal of schizophrenia they reveal themselves as the true, and greatest, source of human anxiety. As patients recover from this illness their residual overload of destructive drives often gets turned against the self, producing clinical depression.

The discovery that each of us has a way to modify the destructive drives was really good news for our human nature. The same kind of shared inner warmth that brought schizophrenics out of their deep withdrawal can relieve pain and suffering in other human crises. The death of a loved one, serious medical illness, wounded pride, all give rise to a surplus of rage that needs to be healed. Perhaps what is really the most important lesson to be learned from the healing of schizophrenics at D.C.General is a spiritual one. The events there strongly suggest a purpose to our existence, namely that we are here for the good of one another.

12

The bureaucrats close in, requiem for an open hospital

Maybe it wasn't a miracle. Paul Barnes had gotten carried away, but deservedly so. He was a hands-on doctor, one of a team of doctors and nurses who did their work down on the wards with real patients who had big problems. It took the visits of two teams of colleagues to make us fully aware of what we had accomplished, for there were no "schizophrenics' at D.C.General Hospital. We had plenty of patients who were schizophrenic by diagnosis, but they no longer functioned as such. Our team was successful because we had enlisted the help of all of our patients and developed a culture in which good human contact was simply a way of life. We weren't miracle workers but we had put together one of the most effective psychiatric hospitals in the world.

One might think that such an achievement would have created permanent job security for all of the personnel involved. It wasn't to be that way. Most of our physicians lost their jobs at D.C. General within the next year, as the open hospital was closed down by a tidal wave of bureaucratic "progress." Then as now there were hands-on doctors, and there were administrative doctors who worked for powerful bureaucratic organizations. It wasn't much of a match between the two groups. The bureaucrats held all the cards.

I should have guessed that John Schultz was up to something when he put a hold on my request to take down the glass security panels from the nursing stations. He had moved up a notch to become Medical Director of the hospital when he left the position of Chief Psychiatrist; and then on to the D.C. Health Department as Chief of Psychiatric Services. There he joined forces with the Director, Dr. Murray Grant, who was a perennial thorn in the side of D.C. General. Together they had cooked up a plan for a bright new tomorrow for the District's psychiatric services, and they had acquired a wealthy co-conspirator in the National Institute of Mental Health. This formidable team of bureaucrats descended on our doctors, nurses, and patients like Byron's well-known wolf on the fold.

The mantra of these brilliant but clinically maladroit federal planners was Community Mental Health Centers, and their bête noire was hospitals. They divided the District up into four quadrants each of which was to be blessed with a CMHC to satisfy its every psychiatric need, including many new ones that were just being dreamed up. The first of these centers was to be established in the old psychiatric pavilion on the grounds of D.C. General Hospital and would bear the nondescript title of the Area C Community Mental Health Center. If you were from Area C, you wouldn't have known it because it existed only on the charts of the planners. The same was true for the other three future CMHC's, Areas A, B and D. The District had sold its psychiatric soul to the NIMH for a mere $500,000 in federal dollars.

There was an interesting condition in the grant that created the Area C-CMHC. No one from the existing psychiatric staff of the D.C. General was to be employed by the new center. John Schultz explained that this apparent aspersion on the quality of our doctors and nurses was the brainchild of the social scientists at the NIMH. He was just playing good cop and bad cop to guarantee his retention of control over the whole operation. Since we had four admitting wards in our hospital, it was a simple enough matter to assign one of these to each of the four new centers to manage their in-patient needs. It looked like a good idea because it would allow our personnel to get even better acquainted with particular neighborhoods in the city. It was also the beginning of our demise. We soon learned that Dr. Schultz wanted the final say as to who would head each ward, and he already had selected an outsider to be the Chief of one of them. At this point he could no longer disguise his intention to take over our program, and I was invited to a meeting in Dr. Murray Grant's office to discuss the relationship between the Area C Center and D.C. General.

John Schultz knew that I was planning to enter full-time private practice in several months so it was not surprising that my resignation date was the first item on the agenda. Dr. Grant insisted that I set the date soon because it was critical to their plans. I suggested that the transition to a new Chief would go very smoothly because either Dr. Novak or Dr. Barnes was well qualified for the job. Then came the bombshell: "We really won't need a Chief Psychiatrist after you leave. The ward medical officers are very experienced and each of them will be the Chief of an in-patient unit that will operate under the supervision of an Area CMHC Director. We have reason to believe that Dr. Steinbach is planning to move Georgetown's residency program over to the VA Hospital, and if he does we will use your salary to fund a panel of hired psychiatrists to cover the night shift for all the units."

I was dumbfounded by the lack of concern, for patients and staff alike, which went into this announcement, as well as the sheer stupidity of two men who probably had higher IQ's than my own. I quieted the urge to accuse them of treating personnel like pawns on a chessboard. Instead I addressed my response to Dr. Grant thinking he would surely see its merit. "You're talking about dismantling what is probably the best public psychiatric hospital in the world," I said, "and destroying it as a functional entity. Wouldn't it be better to keep a place like this as a stable back up for all of the new CMHC's? I think your plan would have a shattering effect on staff morale, which is the key to our success, and it would lead to very uneven levels of care throughout the building. Dr. Novak or Dr. Barnes are both well liked and respected by the entire staff. They could maintain the high standard of care at D.C. General, and would be very supportive of the new centers."

"Well we've been studying this whole thing very carefully," Dr. Grant announced, "and we need a new system of mental health care in the District."

"Yes," John agreed, "things are going to be different. We'll be able to have psychiatrists going into schools and doing preventive mental health work. The centers will enlist the support of local churches to help people with their problems."

"And who will take care of the schizophrenics?" I asked.

"Oh we'll look after them too," said John, with Murray Grant nodding approval. Reading the mix of anger and incredulity on my face John made his final point: "Jim, you've done a good job with D.C. General and you've proven that St. Elizabeth's is no longer needed for the fresh cases of schizophrenia. Of course they still have about 6,000 chronic patients who live there but we won't try to change that until the new area centers are all up and running."

"We'll get to them soon enough," added Murray Grant. "There's going to be a lot of new federal money coming in."

They asked if I could be ready to leave in about a month, and I said, "I'd have to speak with Dr. Steinbach first to see what his plans were for the residency program." Within a half hour I was in Dick Steinbach's office ready to breath fire along with him, and map out a counterattack to keep D.C. General for Georgetown.

"Dick we've got big problems," I began, and got no further.

"John called me already," he said with a rather sour look on his face. "They want you out of there in a month," he continued. "They can't wait to get their hands on your salary so they can hire some psychiatrists to work the night shift."

"We've got to stop him right now," I said. "He's out to do a total takeover."

"It won't do any good," the professor intoned as he lit a cigarette to sooth his own anger. "He's absolutely obsessed with the idea that his new centers will have a prophylactic effect on mental illness, and reduce the need for hospitals."

"But what are they going to do that we're not already doing at D.C.General?" I asked.

"That's exactly the point," Dick said. "I asked John that and he really got angry. I think he's furious with you because you've stolen his thunder and you're making his whole plan look unnecessary. Those centers are supposed to keep sick people in the community and you're doing that better than anyone else in the country. So John and his planners are envious of you and they want to take what you have and put their own name on it. I'm fed up with the whole bunch of them and I don't have the time and the energy to fight with them anymore."

"What about the staff at D.C.General, Dick? How do we protect their jobs?" I asked.

"Well Bill Novak is going to leave soon anyway for the same reason you have to go right now, the time demands of the psychoanalytic institute. I've made up my mind to move the residency program to the VA Hospital and we'll have staff jobs for a couple of them there. As for your nursing staff, none of them will be fired, and they'll probably all end up getting raises with some of that new money John expects to bring in."

It was as simple as that. Both Dick Steinbach and I were willing to let D.C.General go for our own personal reasons: his because he couldn't stand the constant intrusions of bureaucrats into the caring and orderly life of his professorship, and mine because I valued becoming a psychoanalyst so highly that I considered my work with schizophrenics less important. If I had it to do all over again, knowing that the accomplishments of D.C.General have not been replicated elsewhere, I would have chosen to stay and fight on my own, and postponed my psychoanalytic ambitions for another year or two.

It all happened suddenly and there wasn't much time to think. D.C.General had been running so smoothly for the preceding several months that I thought it would either survive as four mini-hospitals or John Schultz would beg Georgetown to resume its stewardship. I never dreamed that it might implode before my very eyes.

Schultz and company, his NIH handlers, did ask me to leave in a month so that they could recruit the night coverage necessitated by Georgetown's withdrawal. My three-week annual vacation had already been scheduled to begin in several days and I would have a week upon return to say good-byes. Meanwhile I invited John Schultz to use my office as his headquarters and he moved in that afternoon.

We shared the space for three days. The man was a human dynamo, grinding out memoranda and swamping the conference table with an endless stream of charts and blueprints. He prowled the building like a nervous cat looking for prey, leaving behind a trail of staff members anxiously pondering his next move. I was never so happy to part from a roommate for a couple of weeks.

To protect the tranquility of my vacation, I had agreed to have one conference call with John Schultz in ten days. His performance ran true to form. After an opening exchange of pleasantries he offered me a new job. He had prevailed on the NIH to allow me to become Chief of the Area C Community Mental Health Center, and to retain my position as Chief Psychiatrist at D.C.General. His exact words were "Jim, you would become the Super Chief." I relayed this information to Dick Steinbach and suggested I would stay on for several months if he were given the power to name my successor. He wasn't moved to compassion for John. "Jim," he said, "The Super Chief is a train that runs out to California, and I wish John would get on it and go there to stay. I'm going to do you and me both a big favor and refuse to even discuss it with him." And that was that.

My return to the hospital was like coming back to a changed homeland after the war. A cloud of depression hung over the building and dampened the spirits of those within. Psychiatrists exchanged gloomy greetings about their latest woes. The happy nursing staff, which had so impressed the visitors from Philadelphia and New York, was somber and jumpy. John Schultz greeted me with a friendly "Hi, Jim," like I hadn't been away, and quickly reported on "a few little problems. We're having some trouble upstairs," he said, "I wonder if you can go up to help out. The new staff from Area C has taken over unit eight but they've been flooded with admissions. They have 53 on the ward right now. (There had been 28 when I left on vacation). I've locked the ward temporarily and they're not accepting any new patients. The other units will have to give them a hand. Meanwhile I was hoping you could pick out some people for emergency transfer to St. Elizabeth's."

I headed upstairs thinking to myself how ironic it was. I was ready to leave D.C. General, and had come to say goodbye, and here at the eleventh hour I'm asked to do the chore that I hate the most, and haven't had to do in years. So be it. I unlocked my way into the unit and saw a dozen patients milling about in front of the locked nursing station. Almost half were in pajamas. They were moving about aimlessly and actually bumping into each other. The potential danger for the outbreak of a fight was clear so that I moved right in and began selecting patients for transfer on sight.

One of the medical students was with me and I tried to do some teaching as we went about our mission. "See that man over there," I said, pointing to a man in pajamas with a blank look on his face. "Let's go talk with him. He may be the first to go." His chart identified him as a former long-term St. Elizabeth's patient who had wandered in off the streets seeking a return to St. E's. We talked for a few moments but the patient was speaking in some form of gibberish. We moved along and I told the student, "You're looking at a classic case of a back-wards patient. They won't even keep him in the receiving building. They'll move him right over to one of the regressed wards." And so I signed his papers for emergency commitment.

Later in the day the student approached me with some startling news. "You know that man we saw this morning, the fellow from the back wards, well he just came up to me and asked me if he could stay here. He sounded O.K. He said he had talked with Dr. Mussenden from the Area C Center and she wanted him to come over there."

The truth flashed across my mind like a bolt of lightening. I had broken my own rule about never judging a patient by their outward appearance, and had made this patient an exception who proved the rule. In this instance at least I knew just what had happened.

Dr. Borinquen Mussenden was a Puerto Rican-American who had trained with me during our first year of residency at D.C. General Hospital. She was a bright person and good doctor who was not yet adapted to our culture, and had a tendency to become very attached to patients. Her application to join the Area C staff had come at a time when they had been unsuccessful in recruiting the type of Ivy League professionals John Schultz and the NIMH had envisioned for their program. John had been concerned that her predilection for holding on to patients might impair her performance in a system geared to the rapid processing of patients.

He may have been right as to her ability to visit the public schools and churches, but for schizophrenic patients she was an excellent physician with a personal warmth ideally suited to their needs. It was instantly clear to me why she had been able to get through whereas I had failed.

We did move about eight patients to St. Elizabeth's that day but the bottle-neck on the Area C ward continued, causing over-crowding on all the wards, and leading to their re-locking not long after my departure. Six months after this time, I was asked by Dick Steinbach to inspect Georgetown's only remaining ward at D.C. General that was now under the direction of the new Area A Community Mental Health Center. It was locked, of course, as were all the other units in the hospital. I looked forward to meeting the young resident who was in charge of the ward, and anticipated that I would have a chance to show him how to make contact with some fresh admissions. We began our time together with a walk through the whole unit just so I could get a taste of the feeling climate there.

It was a horrifying experience. There were no patients milling around, and there was no danger of fights. Quite the opposite. We were looking at 30 detached zombies, mostly in pajamas, not one of who was in any kind of contact with another, or with us. There were no new patients for interview, only stale ones that were over-medicated and awaiting their trip to St. Elizabeth's. It was also a depressing experience and I sensed that the resident doctor, too, was in a state of depression. He certainly had a hopeless attitude about the outlook for his patients.

I told him that I'd like to interview a couple of patients with him to see if I could establish contact with them, and he looked at me like I was demented. "Interview them?" he said, "You can't do that. These patients are too far out of it to interview. It would be a waste of time. But I'll tell you what the trouble is over here. These patients are just too sick to benefit from medications so we're not getting to see how these drugs work. I think our patients need a couple of months of drug therapy at St. E's before medication has any chance to make a difference." I tried to tell him about our experience with the open hospital and now he looked at me like I was delusional. He excused himself saying it was time to begin rounds.

I stopped by Dr. Steinbach's office on my way from the consultation to offer my sympathy. We reminisced about the old days at D.C. General, and then he said, "You know what's happened at D.C. General is the saddest chapter in my career since I've been at Georgetown. It must have been very painful for you to go there today. I'm going to get our residents out of there as soon as I can." And with that we ended our requiem for D.C. General, for it was truly dead as a treatment facility.

The demise of D.C.General marked the beginning of a painful new era for public mental health in the District of Columbia. The folly of closing a caring and very effective hospital for the acutely ill was followed by a frontal assault on St. Elizabeth's Hospital and the evacuation of six thousand of its patients, a majority of who ended up on the streets of D.C. In their haste to open new mental health centers the planners created a social catastrophe. There are now far more people addicted to street drugs, and living on the subway grates, than there are patients in the less crowded new centers. Similar conditions prevail around the rest of the country as we reap the benefits of the emptying out of the state hospitals.

The staff at D.C.General had an amazing capacity to remain connected with their patients after discharge. They took special care of those who had no families of their own, encouraging them to keep in touch with the ward personnel, their doctors, and the excellent clinicians in our psychology and social service departments. They knew that these people were more vulnerable to relapse, and could wind up on the streets without their support. The wonderful new anti-psychotic medications will never banish schizophrenics from the streets unless they are dispensed by people who care enough to get through to them in a personal way. The greatest tragedy in the takeover of D.C.General by bureaucrats is that it caused many of Washington's mentally ill to lose the guardian of their sanity, and only remaining friend, the D.C.General Hospital.

13

Getting through to Julia, an "incurable" schizophrenic

The abrupt eviction of Georgetown from D.C.General terminated my work with schizophrenics for a couple of years. The only use I could make of what we had learned there was by teaching an annual course in schizophrenia at the Baltimore-Washington Institute for Psychoanalysis. I was even beginning to question my memory of the remarkable healing of patients we had seen there. None of the psychiatrists taking my courses had ever seen the same kind of improvement in people who were psychotic. An opportunity to renew my clinical work with a schizophrenic finally arrived before dawn one morning.

Gasoline shortages have a way of bringing people together, and we were in the midst of one at the time. A colleague and I had formed a two-man carpool that took us into downtown Washington at six in the morning. You talk about all kinds of things at that hour and he caught me one morning, still bleary-eyed, with a challenging question. "Jim, I hear you're teaching in your course that schizophrenia is almost always treatable by psychological approaches. Is that true?"

His question awakened me fully like a mental alarm clock going off and I answered with an emphatic "Yes".

"Well, I have a man in treatment", he began, "whose sister has been in a good private hospital for two years for an illness that hasn't gotten any better. The staff there has declared her to be a "process schizophrenic," (an old term that meant the illness had gone beyond the brain to involve other bodily organs and become incurable.) They have advised the family to have her committed to the state hospital. Some of them believe she may also have chronic encephelitis, but in any case they can't help her and they want the family to arrange for her transfer this month. Would you be willing to see her in consultation?"

I paused for a while to think about his question. In almost eight years at D.C. General I had never seen anyone who had been in a state of deep schizophrenic withdrawal for that long. I thought to myself "If a hospital can't get through to her in two years, how am I going to do it in one meeting? And besides, the hospital is up in Philadelphia so it would take a whole day out of my busy life."

My colleague went on, as I weighed an answer, with an interesting detail about the woman's sickness. "Her breakdown occurred when her first baby, a little girl, was only eight months old. She hasn't seen the child since then because she became so disturbed during family visits, they were afraid for the safety of the baby."

I had realized the consultation would be a good learning opportunity for myself, and a source of fresh clinical material for my course. But his comment about the mother and her baby did it. "Tom, that's just plain wrong," I answered. "How can anyone help a patient get back into the real world if they don't permit contact with the most important part of the real world in that person's life? Yes, I'll go see the patient. Tell her brother to call me."

Her brother came in for a meeting, which he began with a down-to-earth clinical summary. "I think they just got tired of treating Julia, and they can't stand her anymore because she's such a mess. She scratches and rubs her face and neck to where they're just covered with open sores, and she pulls out clumps of her hair. She's on antibiotics all the time because these things get infected, and I think they're afraid she'll get a staph infection, and cause an epidemic in the whole place. They've given her Thorazine and Haldol (a heavy-duty tranquilizer) in large doses, but nothing seems to help her illness. Besides that she never remembers the names of anyone there, and she can't even remember conversations she's had with the staff a minute later. Some of them think she must have encephalitis because she has no memory and her mind just doesn't work right."

I asked if there was anyone at all on the staff with whom she was able to speak. He responded, "Well, yes, there is. Her name is Betty and she's just a plain country girl. She lives way out in the county on a farm with her parents. I think maybe she's kind of attached to them like sis was to mom and dad before she met her husband." I asked if he knew what they talked about, and he replied, "No, I really don't. I guess maybe they talk about her farm. Sis used to say she'd like to live on a farm someday." I told him that I wanted to be sure that Betty could be there on the day of my visit.

He then offered some thoughts about the origin of his sister's illness. "We used to kid about sis because she was so close to mom. You've got to know my mother. She tries to run every detail of everybody's life, and the rest of us just stay away from her, but not sis. Mom did all her thinking for her, and sis liked it that way. When she met Vince (her husband), he had a strong personality too, like Mom, and he took over her life, but she still managed to see mom most every day. After they got married, Vince was transferred to Chicago for an auditing job. They moved right away and it nearly killed my sister because she missed mom so much. To make it worse her husband had to travel a lot so she was alone a good bit on weekends. I think she cried every time I called and she was furious about the whole thing because she thought Vince could have stayed in the Washington area.

Then she got pregnant and that helped in some ways because she really wanted to have a baby, but it made her even angrier because mom wasn't around and wouldn't be able to come after the baby's birth. She had a little girl and was depressed at first, but then she really got all caught up in being a good mother and was o.k. for a while. Vince had a chance to come back to Washington about a month before her breakdown but he turned it down because he thought he could move ahead faster in Chicago. That made her boil over like nothing I've ever seen and to top it off he had to be away on a couple of trips to the West Coast. She took him out to the airport for one and on the way back she began to hear voices urging her to kill herself. She went to her next-door neighbor and her speech was incoherent so they took her to the state hospital, where they admitted her. Next day she went to another psychiatric hospital downtown where she was mute, and she stayed there a month. She couldn't talk at all to the doctors or nurses there, or even to Vince, but a couple of times when we were alone she talked to me a little.

After that they moved her to the hospital in Philadelphia, which was not too far from mom, and Vince got a job in Washington where his sister was able to help out with the little girl. Sis started to talk again up there, and Vince and mom are able to visit, but they have funny visiting hours. Vince is allowed to come once a week for a half-hour, and mom can only visit every other week for ten minutes. That's because sis really goes wild after mom leaves. Anyhow I just thought if she hadn't moved to Chicago she would have been all right, but now I don't know if she's ever going to be normal again."

I made arrangements for the consultation with her husband, and he basically confirmed her brother's account of the illness. He regretted his decision to remain in Chicago so long and was beginning to feel despair about his wife's prospects for recovery. He made it very clear that he was committed to the marriage and would stand by his wife whatever the outcome. He spoke enthusiastically about their daughter, now two-and-a-half, and didn't question the decision to keep her from visiting her mother because his wife seemed unaware of her existence. He added the worrisome detail that he had tried to have his wife evaluated at a university hospital in Philadelphia but her admission had been put on hold for fear of a contagious staph infection.

The day of our meeting dawned gloomy and gray with foreboding clouds of rain above. It almost seemed as though the outside gloom had penetrated and pervaded the dayroom except for one cheery alcove that Betty had reserved for us. She shook my hand warmly, while Julia shook it not at all. Julia was indeed a mess with open sores the size of a quarter covering her face, neck and arms. She was extremely obese, her eyes were glazed, and her pupils fixed at pinpoint aperture. We were at the zero level of contact.

She sported a bright red scarf that I asked about immediately, think-ing it must have been a Christmas present. I felt that she would surely be aware of such a colorful piece of reality, and how it had come into her possession, but her response was a toneless, "I don't know." And that's how it went for the next five minutes as I tried in vain to engage her in a present interest. I stumbled about in darkness touching on breakfast, lunch, Betty, the dayroom, the rain clouds, all to no avail. A long forgotten poem from high school, Francis Thompson's "Hound of Heaven" ran through my mind. Even as I pursued my efforts with Julia, I was pondering the lines, "I fled Him down the nights, and down the days, I fled Him down the labyrinthine ways of my own mind." The analyst in me intruded with the observation: "She's running away from you all right, and you're getting lost in the labyrinths of her mind. But if she's the runner then you must think you're God and that you can cure anybody." I laughed to myself at this sudden intrusion of grandiose fantasy, aware that I felt the kind of hopelessness about Julia that could have used some help from God.

Her brother had described her as a good mother to her infant daughter, and I had planned to discuss early visits with the child if we should decide to transfer her to a new hospital under my care. With some trepidation I raised this possibility with Julia (and Betty), and her response was a flat "I don't have children." Looking surprised, her companion said, "But you were showing me some pictures of her just last week. I'll get them from your locker."

Until that point, I felt I had had almost no meaningful contact with my future patient. I can recall looking at her pinpoint and motionless pupils and thinking, "I'm completely shut out. There must be a person in there, but she's way down deep inside." Betty's return with the pictures really didn't seem to make any difference. The patient perused them with the same total indifference that she had for the rest of the world. There was one brief moment when she evinced a kind of sudden and shocking contact with reality, and that was when Betty commented that she looked "so slim back then" (before her hospitalization). She winced in painful awareness of the fact that she had gained over 100 pounds since that time.

As I prepared to leave, I felt quite depressed. She hadn't reacted to the pictures with any sign of realization that she had a daughter, and my words about moving her to another hospital appeared to have fallen on deaf ears. I wondered why we hadn't reached a warming point, that wonderful moment at D.C.General when patients began to show a little life. I had tried all my best leads for one without success. Suddenly she looked in my direction and seized my hand, squeezing it gently. "When can I come to the new hospital?" was all that she said, but the compact had been sealed. Her family called later with "remarkable news, she's remembering something for the first time. She remembers your name, and she knows that she's going to meet you in the new hospital on Monday."

On my way home from the consultation I stopped off at the Georgetown University Hospital to tell Dick Steinbach about my interesting patient. Chatting with his secretary, I found out that their new inpatient unit was only half-full and looking for patients. When he emerged, I greeted him with a thought that had suddenly occurred to me. Describing Julia's condition, I asked if we might bring her into Georgetown's new psychiatric ward instead of the hospital that was holding a bed for her.

"Dick," I said, "I plan to see her every day for as long as necessary to bring her out of her psychotic withdrawal. I hope she'll be able to manage a reunion with her daughter in about two weeks. She would be a marvelous teaching case for the residents and students." I could see from the look on his face that the answer was no. "Jim," he finally replied, "It just won't work. Our nursing staff is really quite inexperienced and they wouldn't be able to handle someone like that. I'll be surprised if you can keep her where she's going. She really does sound like a process schizophrenic. It's too bad your old program at D.C. General isn't around anymore. Your staff could have helped her, but they're scattered all around town now. We really don't have any good hospitals for difficult schizophrenics in Washington." And so it was that Julia and I came to the new hospital early on Monday, ready to begin our journey together.

In our program at D.C. General Hospital, once good human contact was established, it was almost always followed by the patient's continued greater degree of involvement in the real world. With Julia, that was not the case. Her arrival on a general hospital psychiatric ward was greeted with consternation by the nursing staff, who had never seen a patient in such deep withdrawal. Her lack of memory for any and every interaction with staff raised the familiar specter of encephalitis, and her self-inflicted wounds were incomprehensible and disgusting. According to hospital regulations she could only stay for 90 days. Most of the nurses expected her to leave for the State Hospital long before then, and the rest felt she would certainly go there on day 91. Making contact was a fresh challenge each day.

I had given Julia's mother permission to come outside the regular visiting hours, which meant, in effect, that she could be there at any hour of the day for any length of time. She more than took advantage of this latitude, she camped in. In my first meeting with her, she was extremely hostile and suspicious, displaying an almost violent hatred for Julia's husband. The words "that bastard" came up at least five times in her opening comments about him as she gradually worked her way around to her conviction that he was a rapist. Over time I recognized that my patient's mother suffered from chronic paranoid schizophrenia and a pathologic preoccupation with the danger of rape, which even then caused her to hover protectively over her daughter. They spent hours together playing cards and consuming enormous quantities of diet coke. Whenever staff members raised the question of encephalitis I would tell them to ask her mother about Julia's excellent skills as a card player.

Our daily visit took place shortly after breakfast so that its timing was reliable and expectable, and there was a ready opening topic regarding the items on the breakfast menu. Initially Julia seemed little more accessible than in our very first meeting, although one of the nurses reported that she had begun to inquire about the time each morning. When asked why she wanted to know she said, "Because my doctor will be coming soon." This anticipatory interest was not in evidence when we met.

During the first week the interview scenarios had a monotonous and boring similarity. The breakfast colloquy would be followed by a review of the luncheon choices and then some discussion about diet Cokes and card games that she was enjoying with her mother. Eventually I would introduce the topic of a visit from her daughter, only to be told that she had no children. Again, we would look at the pictures that were now kept in her bedside stand. I would remind her that we had talked about her daughter coming just yesterday, but even then she seemed not to acknowledge her existence.

After several days, I chanced by the hospital gift shop on my way to see her. There, on a shelf, was a tiny yellow convertible car that attracted my attention. Julia had owned an old convertible before her move to Chicago, and both her husband and brother called it her best friend. She had named it Millie after her best human friend. (She had also bestowed the same name on her daughter.) I bought the little car and gave it with the suggestion that it would be nice to have a present for her daughter to play with on her visit. She obviously enjoyed receiving the gift, and subsequently kept it on top of her bedside stand. She would pick it up and look at it whenever we discussed the impending reunion, but she continued to deny that such an event could actually happen because she "had no children." It wasn't until the day before the meeting, which was set for the end of her second week in the hospital, that Julia began to show a kind of marginal awareness that the event was going to take place.

My drive to the hospital that Sunday morning was the occasion for a strange admixture of feelings. Bright hopes for a successful family visit were intermingled with forebodings of failure. Julia's interest in the whole project had progressed from totally non-evident to highly questionable. Would she be withdrawn, inaccessible, or even wildly psychotic? What about the impact on her little daughter? There had already been some significant murmuring among the nurses about it. When we finally received word that her family had arrived in the hospital lobby, both doctor and patient were bracing themselves for the unknown.

The lobby had been selected as the most hospitable site for a child's visit, and Julia and I had about a minute together while we waited for the elevator. To my amazement Julia's face had come to life with an expressiveness I had never seen. Looking me right in the eye she said, "Dr. Ryan, I'm scared, really scared. What if she doesn't recognize me? It's been so long. And what do I say to her?"

To which I replied, "Julia, you were a good mother to her when she was a baby. For that reason I think that deep down she's going to know who you are. And for the same reason, you'll know just what to say to her." And then we were in the lobby where her daughter raced towards her with shouts of "Mommy, Mommy." Julia hoisted her aloft for one big hug while they showered each other with kisses.

Julia had been transformed into a completely normal person. During the next half-hour, she smiled and radiated her approval as her daughter performed innumerable tricks for her. She asked her questions, and responded to her daughter's queries with genuine warmth. And when her youngster's enthusiastic play with the convertible threatened the decorum of the lobby, she set firm and appropriate limits. She was indeed a good mother, and for those 30 minutes without a trace of schizophrenia.

On our elevator ride back to the unit, I had expected that we would be able to share some of the sweet memories of the visit. How wrong I was. Once again a total transformation occurred, and I was with the Julia of day one of our acquaintance. During the week, as we prepared for the next visit, she had no memory whatsoever of the one that had just transpired. Again, she had "no children," and again the photographs seemed to move her not at all. On subsequent Sundays the same radical shifts between Julia, the patient, and Julia, the mother, took place. We were soon to learn the reason why.

For the first six weeks, we were able to meet every day, but now our relationship faced a critical test. A family holiday was coming up that would take me away for four days. I decided to bring it up with Julia about a week in advance, and did so early in one of our meetings that were now taking place in an office on the ward. As she started to respond, her speech became slurred. She stammered, almost choked on her own words, and finally lapsed into an infantile babble. I commented on how difficult it must be for her to face the prospect of my being away for four days, when we had been working so closely together every day. She said yes, and regained at least a limited capacity to speak in halting phrases for the rest of the session. When we arose from our chairs to leave the office, she stood there, frozen in place, motionless and mute. She was clearly watching me, almost slyly, out of the corner of her eye. Again I commented on the pain my announcement had caused, and I added that, "It has also stirred up a lot of rage for you, so much that you're straining every muscle to keep it under control." Her eyes said yes, she nodded in agreement and proceeded to walk slowly to her room.

On the following morning she approached her favorite nurse with the usual inquiry about the time, and the latter asked, "Are you still angry with Dr. Ryan because he's going away next week?" Whereupon she exploded with rage, and shrieked, "No, I'm not angry with my damned doctor. He can go to Hell. I could just tear him to bits. I'd like to bite his head off." The nurse had taken the heat from her boiling rage.

When I arrived on the ward a few minutes later, Julia was withdrawn with a marked flattening of her feelings. I said, "You seem very distant from me right now, but I was told that you had some very intense feelings a few minutes ago out in the hall." Much to my surprise she smiled, and then repeated the details of her encounter with the nurse word-for-word and with relish. She added, "I wanted to grind you up with my teeth and spit you out." Over the next few days she was to heap additional verbal coals on my head about the vacation, but she also began to see dimly that the rage that had overcome her with the announcement of my trip had some connection with rage attacks she had been having when she first entered the hospital in Philadelphia.

She knew she had been furious and almost "boiling over" at times before her breakdown in Chicago but she had no memories about her hospitalization there. In Philadelphia, she had begun to have visits by her mother and husband, but they quickly became very painful and generated rage because of the interminably long period she would have to endure before the next visit. She found that by withdrawing she could "wipe these things out" of her mind immediately after the departure of her family, and thereby reduce her pain and distress. She was able to "vaporize them", to mentally destroy them so entirely that she had no memory whatsoever of their visits, not even any fleeting visual images of her mother or husband. They no longer existed. While this process was going on, she found that the comings and goings of all human beings in her daily life were also so painful that she "blanked them out" entirely. They became non-happenings. I asked if she ever thought about Betty and she said, "Who?" She was without any kind of mental picture she could connect with the name.

There were no further episodes of catatonia, and Julia was able to remember me during my absence, talking each day with staff about where I was, and what I was doing. We had agreed ahead of time that she would do this, and she actually began to look forward to these conversations. Her capacity for recollection of interactions with staff returned, and more importantly, she could now remember and talk about her absent family. It was no longer necessary to use a magical memory cut-off switch to control her rage.

When I returned, Julia was ready for a trial on her first weekend pass, and first visit to her new home. A vigorous staff debate followed my declared intention to issue such a pass because most of the nurses still found her to be "totally psychotic" in their contacts with her. The two with whom she had been discussing my absence were in full agreement with the trip home, even though Julia was still gouging out new holes in her skin occasionally.

Julia's visit was successful enough to repeat it on each of the remaining weekends of hospitalization. These visits were marked by a kind of child-like dependency on her husband and good contact with her daughter. Once back in the hospital she still looked and behaved like a back-wards patient except in her interactions with a few of the nurses whom she liked. We were nearing the 90-day deadline and a decision had to be made whether to transfer her to another in-patient ward, or send her home to participate in a day care program. Her husband set four requirements for her return: she must be able to manage her own medication, prepare her daughter to attend nursery school each morning, learn to use public transportation, and limit visitation with her mother to once a week. Any one of these had looked like it might be an impossibility for her but Julia set to work on all four tasks and was discharged to her home on the 89th day.

Initially she came for outpatient psychotherapy three times a week, and later twice weekly, always by bus. Her debut in the day care center was marked by staff apprehension about her ability to function in a group of people who were obviously much less regressed than herself. After about a month there, she was seen by a well-known and well-respected Washington psychiatrist in a peer review of my treatment of her. When he had completed his examination he said, "Jim, why are you treating her with psychotherapy? She's a process schizophrenic. You can't help her." Julia had successfully fended off every effort on his part to establish some warmth with her, and he was angry. I had heard those words before, but now I knew they were wrong.

Julia graduated from the day care center in about three months and began a part-time job that eventually required six hours of office work each weekday. By the end of a year, she had weaned herself off all medication and had healed a major ego wound by losing 100 pounds of weight. Her skin lesions were about 80% healed so that she could comfortably take her daughter to a swimming pool, but she was still gouging her skin at times.

We were meeting once a week then, on Saturday mornings. One bright fall day when Mother Nature was beckoning all humans with a come hither look, she arrived at my office with her husband and daughter. All three were talking enthusiastically about the supplies they needed to buy that day for Halloween. As she entered the sterile confines of my consultation room, Julia could see Vince and their daughter skipping out the door, hand-in-hand, on their way to make the purchases. We sat down, and she began to dig her nails into her skin, while looking at me with sustained eye contact. On every previous occasion in which she had carried out this ritual in my presence, she had done so in a kind of impenetrable, glassy-eyed detachment from reality. My efforts to discuss this symptom with her had gotten nowhere. But that day we were clearly in very good contact.

I said, "I can see that you're aware of what you're doing today, and that you don't mind if I too am aware of it. So now we can begin to talk with each other about what's happening." Looking at the arm, which she was now rubbing vigorously with her thumb and scratching with her index finger, she said, "You're down there and so is Vince and Millie. Soon you'll all be ground to bits and pieces and I'll blow you away like dust."

I said, "You're so enraged by my keeping you from your family when they're having fun that you have to wipe out the whole scene and get rid of all of us. But the only one who is going to suffer from your rage is yourself. You're being very cruel to yourself right now." She sat bolt upright and looked stunned as though a new perception of herself had finally gotten through. "Yes," she said, "I'm making myself the victim and this has got to stop."

Her terrible attacks on her own flesh ended that day and for a number of sessions she continued to work on memories in which she relived and verbally expressed her outrage about the cruel restrictions her mother had imposed on her play both with other children and when alone. As more and more detail emerged about her mother's strange behavior, Julia began to see that her mother had been suffering from a psychotic illness throughout her childhood. Her attitude towards her mother shifted from one of fury to one of pity, and a genuine warmth in their relationship became possible for the first time. One of Julia's biggest fears after the reunion with her daughter had been that she might damage her by holding on to her too tightly. As she broke the bondage with her mother she became more relaxed with her daughter, and able to enjoy the little one's increasing independence. Julia had completed the incorporation of a kinder and warmer mother, a female version of Dr. Ryan, into her own make-up, and her treatments stopped at this point except for brief problem-solving sessions every three or four months. About two years later, she came in one evening to ask if I saw any problem in her having another baby, or maybe even several more babies. I didn't and she did just that, raising a family of four healthy children. She has had no recurrence of schizophrenic illness.

Getting through to Julia had only been possible because a tiny bit of warm feeling about her daughter had survived the massive withdrawal that wiped out her conscious awareness that she had any offspring. That little flame of warmth, though buried deeply within her shattered and disorganized self, was available for a kindling reaction with a doctor's concern about her. Our inner warmth is the hallmark of our human nature, it is the "something special" about being human that draws us to one another. Perhaps the greatest lesson we can learn from Julia's story is that our capacity for love survives, even when we are completely over-run by hateful feelings.

The understanding that such a kernel of love had to be somewhere within her motivated me to keep with the topic of her daughter even though she kept pushing it away. My outreach finally got through to this loving portion of her inner self and drew a response of warmth from her in the form of a gentle hand squeeze. It is interesting that she was only able to express her good feeling in this way, considering that the chief outlet for her destructive drives had been the use of her hands as claws to gouge her own flesh. The power of her loving instincts to modify her destructive drives was certainly operating at an appropriate location.

Getting through to someone usually refers to the transmission of ideas or feelings from one person to another. With schizophrenics, a much richer assortment of mental supplies must be exchanged in order to restore psychological life. In our first meeting, getting through to Julia meant bringing her warmth, hope, trust, some rational thought and a selective memory. On our way to meet her daughter, there was a much greater visual and emotional sharing that imparted self-confidence and self-control.

For Julia our daily experiences of getting through established a psychological umbilical cord on which she was dependent for the sustenance of her emotional life. When I told her that I would be away for four days, she reacted with an outpouring of rage towards me consistent with her perception that I was shutting down her lifeline. It was a repetition of the traumatic separation in Chicago from her mother and husband. But the process of getting through continued to supply her with the resources necessary to modify her rage so that she was able to emerge quickly from her catatonic state. The intervention, in which she was able to use her doctor's and her own loving energies to tame her primitive rage, was a major healing event. It allowed her to regain her memory for the comings and goings of other people in her life, greatly strengthening her ties to the real world.

The final event in Julia's healing came when she signaled, in a moment of eye-to-eye contact that she was ready for an experience of getting through. Once again her destructive drives were in ascendancy but she herself was their most immediate victim. They had been set-off by an appointment with me that interfered with her enjoyment of two people much more important than I, her husband and daughter. Her self-destructiveness had been obvious to everyone except herself. Then, in a flash, she was able to see it because it was coming from someone so close as to be a part of herself. It was the right time for her to have this insight. She had prepared herself through two years of close contact with a less abrasive mother-substitute.

The very essence of all healing is the mobilization of our loving energies, with help from the outside, to confront and modify the destructive drives that lie dormant in all of us but seek to assert themselves from time-to-time. Our inner warmth is a great human asset, possessed by all, which can be used to mitigate suffering in others. When we make our healing power available for this purpose, it actually grows in strength because of the loving feedback it generates. The consequent enhancement of our inner warmth serves to further protect us from our own destructive drives.

Julia's healing reveals how much in common psychotherapy can have with a platonic love relationship. Was there an actual exchange of warmth going on throughout our meetings? Was there a two-way street for the delivery of healing energies in both directions? Let's look at the record. Julia's little squeeze of my hand just before our first parting rescued me from depression and sent me on my way with a good feeling that gradually caused a marked increase in self-confidence. After I dropped in on Dr. Steinbach I found myself unexpectedly suggesting that I would use her treatment as an on-going teaching case for the resident physicians and medical students at Georgetown. Dick said "You've certainly come a long way in what you expect to accomplish with regressed patients." I didn't tell him that my assessment of her case was based on the vote of confidence given in Julia's warm handshake and her decision to change hospitals.

When she arrived in the "new hospital" I met with a wave of resentment and outright criticism from the nursing staff for bringing in someone whom they deemed "inappropriate" for their setting. She seemed to be totally oblivious to her surroundings or anything else in the outside world for that matter. But she did badger them with repeated questions about the time of day until they finally asked her why this was such an important concern. Her answer "Because my doctor will be coming soon" was spoken with such reverence that it has been a reminder to me ever since of how special it is to be a doctor, and how great a responsibility we have to try to meet our patients needs. Her simple answer told the nurses all they needed to know about the value and necessity for her presence in the hospital.

My purchase of the toy car may have done more for me than it did for Julia. I didn't think of it at the time but this spontaneous gesture came right out of the golden years of my training at the Beth Israel Hospital in Boston. It was known there as a "manipulation" and consisted in taking advantage of a flawed part in a patient's make-up to gain their greater cooperation. I knew that Julia had lots of abandonment anxiety and I gave her this reminder of a joyful era in her life to help her to keep me in her mind while I was away. It became perhaps the most favored object in her environment, occupying a prominent place on her bedside stand. It also served me as a daily reminder of an important time in my own development as a psychiatrist, when we were working with uncooperative medical patients at Beth Israel.

The experience of finally learning the meaning of why she gouged out craters on her skin struck me as a reward for our two years together. She was sharing a precious secret that allowed her to sever her connection with a psychotic mother, and to complete her treatment. The intimacy of shared secrets is the staff of life for psychiatrists. Julia's was an especially meaningful one. I came out of her treatment as a better doctor.

14

Psychosurgery for suicidal depressions

Depression has to be the most common of mental afflictions since it is a condition that all of us experience at least in low dosage at one moment or another almost every day. When it becomes intense and long lasting, it is also the most painful disturbance of the mind. Self-love is then lost and self-loathing rules the day. In one of his greatest papers, Freud compared the normal process of mourning with the pathological state of melancholia, an old term for any type of depression that became long lasting, with a progressive downhill course. He showed how a beloved person, who has been lost by death, or even a lost ideal, can be taken into the self, and is then pilloried by all the hatred that is engendered by the loss.

The victims of this relentless illness are tormented by self-accusations of inadequacy that deprive them of restful sleep and awaken them prematurely to face another terrible day. They lose their appetite for food, eating and other vital functions become burdensome, and their bodies undergo a dramatic shrinkage. Crying spells may be frequent and beyond control, the powers of concentration are lost, and finally death may be contemplated as the only escape route. In their broken-down state they present themselves to others as pathetic creatures that are helpless and not even up to the slightest tasks of daily living. For this reason they might also seem to be harmless, but they have a powerful underlying rage that fuels a violent force by which they tear themselves to shreds. They are thus a constant menace to themselves, they feel physically worn out by their own aggression, and suicide is an all too frequent consequence. Barring a fatal outcome, almost all will recover from this devastating illness, although they will remain more vulnerable to recurrence than the next person.

The term melancholia has disappeared from our diagnostic code-books but full blown, serious depressions with the danger of suicide still account for more hospital admissions than any other form of mental ill-ness. They require vigorous treatment with the good anti-depressant drugs now available and will usually achieve full recovery. Some people with serious depressions become drug resistant and remain suicidal. They may go through three or four changes of psychiatrists in a fruitless search for the right drug. These patients need the healing intervention of another human being to lead them out of an illness where medica-tion has failed. Over the years I have treated about twenty such patients successfully, and it took me quite a while to realize that a special kind of getting through with inner warmth was going on. One evening, as I was preparing to lead a seminar in depression for a small group of psychia-trists, it all came together in my mind around the following three patients.

Rosemary was a fifty-year-old single woman, and computer special-ist, whose capacity for daily overtime work was highly valued by her employer. She had become depressed shortly after the start of a four week vacation with fears that she was "just not good enough" for her job, and would lose it. Her depression had a rapid downhill course with severe feelings of worthlessness, some suicidal thoughts, loss of appetite, frequent crying spells, and a disturbing insomnia of three weeks dura-tion. Her family doctor had prescribed two anti-depressants and four different types of sleeping medicines to no avail. She became housebound and finally developed the delusion that someone was trying to kill her with poison gas. When her physician referred her for consultation he commented that she and her elderly mother were the last occupants of the old family home, and the latter had been bedridden with congestive heart failure for much of the past several months.

During our first meeting, she began in a detached way to describe how she had noticed the poison gases on a visit to her office and suspected a plot among her coworkers to kill her. She was afraid she might become a victim of such an attack anytime she was outside her own home. She gave a disjointed account of her reasons for feeling worthless, almost as if she were lost amid a welter of disturbing experiences. She would go from one to another, the only recurrent theme being her insomnia and consequent incapacitation for work. She alluded to her mother's illness briefly, saying that she had begun to notice deterioration in her condition during the vacation. In this regard she cited the presence of urinary and fecal odors in her bedroom. (Perhaps these were the real poison gases.) Her mother's increasing difficulties in traveling from her room to the kitchen downstairs had disabled her for preparing meals.

I asked her to tell me exactly what it was like when she was trying to go to sleep and she told me that her whole body was tired, but she just could not find a comfortable position. She would shift her head one way or another, move her arms and legs, turn from back to stomach, so that no part of her was relaxed. I felt impelled to say something. What came out was unplanned and quickly evolved into a spontaneous utterance that had a life of its own. I said, "If you begin to feel that way again tonight, I want you to get out of bed and walk down the hallway, quietly, past your mother's room, and go downstairs to the kitchen. Open the refrigerator and pour yourself a glass of milk. Warm the milk, but carefully. Not too hot, you want it to be just right. When you drink the milk, it will feel good inside, and it will be easier to relax and fall asleep." She agreed with this plan, and I concluded with, "Can you come over tomorrow morning so we can talk some more. How about 11:30?"

It worked. The patient arrived promptly at 11:30 the next morning with a smile on her face. Not a great big smile, but enough to tell me ahead of time that she had slept. She was enormously pleased with this accomplishment and able to talk about her worries and low feelings in much less frantic tones. She returned to work on schedule in two days. We met twice a week for a few weeks, then once a week for several more, and once a month for about five times. She was able to take the step of placing her mother in a nursing home and began to date a man regularly for the first time in her life.

Early in Rosemary's consultation, I had thought that it might be necessary to fill out emergency commitment papers for the state hospital. As she described her efforts to get to sleep, I could feel the agony of her tortured body inside myself. She had succeeded in placing the true object of her self-torture, her disabled mother, inside of me for safekeeping. I had only one thing in mind as I began my response and that was to get her out of that bed and find something to do that would be soothing. Words tumbled out ahead of thought, soon followed by the flash of a dream-like image of a mother holding her toddler's upraised hand and helping her to walk. We were already downstairs, having tiptoed past her mother's room, when the idea of warm milk occurred. What better gift from a soothing mother? Her damaged and disabled mother was now the bountiful one of old, a reliable protector whose presence made it possible to face the fearful task of falling asleep in order to reap its restful pleasures. Over several months, my patient progressed from walking hand-in-hand to taking some very important life-steps on her own, with the steady approval of her physician. Hope had been restored and the nightmare of delusions and despair was over.

In the next few years I saw two more patients with severe depressions who hadn't benefited at all from any of the good anti-depressants then available. After several months each of them had reached the hospital in a suicidal state (one after an almost successful attempt.) As in Rosemary's case where I had intuitively made a blatantly hypnotic suggestion, each of these patients responded to an intuitive and highly unusual behavior on my part in our first meeting. I played my first game of shuffleboard in the hospital with the man who had almost killed himself, and I gave my second patient's wife a very sharp reprimand in front of him when she suggested, reasonably enough, that he quit his job so they could live on his pension.

My patient who had attempted suicide had just come off the intensive care unit, was pacing in his room and almost jumping out of his skin with anxiety when I suggested the game of shuffleboard. At the conclusion of this contest, which he won, he gave me a look of admiration and gratitude that I'll never forget. In each subsequent meeting he reported on fresh accomplishments that marked his rapid rise out of depression. I learned later that his depression had begun after a visit with his father on the family farm in which he realized that his father's strength was ebbing so fast that his final days were near. He reminisced about a number of physical games he and his father had played while he was growing up. He also complained about missing his son and "best golfing partner" who was then in a remote post overseas with the State Department.

The third patient was really at death's door when he arrived at the hospital malnourished and dehydrated. He had a delusion that his stomach had stopped working so that he was in danger of choking on food and water. He was totally unable to care for himself and his wife had taken over his daily life quite appropriately and completely. She suddenly thrust a statement of resignation from his job in front of him, saying, "You'll have to sign this so we can begin collecting your pension."

At that point I rose from my chair, and with a stern look at his wife I snapped, "Now wait just a minute. Your husband has been very depressed but that's no reason for him to resign from his job. He's had a wonderful career with the foundation and we have to figure out why he's become depressed, to help him get over it, and get back to work." Even as I made this strongly authoritarian statement I wondered whether I had completely misread my patient, and suggested a goal he couldn't even begin to think about. A nurse present at my first meeting with the couple later asked me "Why did you speak with her so harshly? That man is never going to be able to work again. He'll be lucky if he gets out of here alive."

I concluded the meeting by telling his wife I would discuss the treatment plan with her right after her husband and I had a chance to meet on the ward. I saw him there a few minutes later and he mumbled the words "Thank you, doctor". He began eating and drinking with my encouragement, and started on a course of steady improvement that led to full recovery and a return to work in five weeks.

In the course of our meetings, as I was exploring for possible causes for the onset of his depression, he said "You know, doctor, what I think has been bothering me more than anything else this year has been the death of my father. He outlived my mother and died at eighty-nine, but he was still a powerful man, never to be crossed. He made me go to college even though none of my friends went there, and I relied on his advice for any big decisions I had to make. I didn't like my mother very much as a kid. She was always jumping all over me with criticisms, but my father could really put her in her place."

One Friday evening I was taking a nap in anticipation of teaching a seminar in depression to a small group of psychiatrists. A psychoanalyst's own couch is the perfect place to catch a restful twenty minutes, and I do it all the time when there is a mental challenge coming up. On this occasion I was also doing a quick review of a number of my patients who had had a sudden upward turn in their depressions, and these three stood out. I found myself thinking about them in some detail when I saw something that made me jump up from the couch and say "Wow!" In each instance, I had done something that was absolutely "not me", not just an uncharacteristic action, but a one of a kind happening without precedent or repetition. I realized that in each case my unusual behavior had been critical to their development of new hope.

The clear meaning of these "not me" experiences was that the patient had actually taken over a portion of my own self and was putting it to his own advantageous usage by the process of "projective identification." Melanie Klein first described this phenomenon as a way of dealing with a severe emotional overload. By this mental mechanism, a person is able to take a troubled part of himself or herself and inject it into someone else who is then moved into an action called an "enactment", that is beneficial to the one distressed. The phenomenon of enactment is another example of the many ways in which our loving energies can be deployed for the good of one another. My depressed patients had been taking out their fury at the terrible loss involved in their parents' deaths on themselves. More specifically, they were ripping and tearing at the part of themselves occupied by their parents. They had almost succeeded in killing off the mental representations of their parents even though we all need their abiding internal presence throughout life as a source of security and good feelings.

The depression, despair and agitation caused by the near destruction of such a basic part of themselves got under my skin and impelled me to do something. In the "not me" behavior, I became one of the old, beloved parents, now recovered from the damage of the depressive process, empathic in their hour of need, and powerful enough to rescue them in just the right way from the grip of depression. They had been able to eject the depressive nucleus of a battered parent into me, moving me to take a spontaneous and intuitive action in which I became the good parent of old.

To look a bit further at these three cases, they too were suffering from an overload of the same kind of raw destructive drives seen in the illness of Julia. They were really nearing the end of the road in their self-destruction, and had already almost demolished that inner lifeline we get from parental love. But they had a last chance for survival and that was to find someone strong enough to contain their aggression and loving enough to heal it. Those qualities are usually assigned to doctors as part of the positive transference phenomenon described by Freud. Doctors aren't the only ones who can heal in this unique way. A member of the clergy, a good friend, or a loyal family member could carry out the same operation. And indeed it is an operation in the truest medical sense of the word. It is a form of psychosurgery in which a diseased part of the mind, a relentlessly progressive pathological process endangering life, is removed through an intimate exchange with another person in whom it gets healed. It is then returned to the patient in a healthy state.

Getting through to depressed patients whose illness was beyond the reach of medication was guided by a doctor's intuitive perception that their relentless attacks on themselves had damaged their loving ties to their parents. Having located this deep wound to the psyche it was possible to remove it from the patient and bring it into the doctor where it took over his very self, and transformed it into a healthy version of one of the parents. The ability of very depressed people to summon forth such help probably came from a psychological immune system developed early in life. Infants in the throes of abandonment rage are repeatedly rescued by a timely dosage with parental love. The ancient memory that such magical rescues can happen allows the very depressed to keep trying even when total hopelessness draws nigh. In any case, we have here another example of a loving resource within our human nature that helps us to act for the good of one another.

15

The repair of lifelong anger

How do we deal with people who are openly abusive toward us, even or perhaps especially in our very first meeting? There are some whose intense anger and destructive urges are so volatile that they spill out quite spontaneously. Psychiatrists have a diagnostic term for many of them that we tend to use more in disdain than with appropriate medical concern. They are called "borderlines", which means borderline personality disorder, and implies a weakness in their personality structure.

Al, a forty-two year old salesman, was a "borderline." He arrived at my office ten minutes late on a referral by his lawyer. He had been ordered to have psychiatric consultation by a judge as part of a plea agreement in which a charge of assault and battery was to be dropped. He told me about an encounter with his landlord in which he had threatened to punch his nose, but only "shoved him around a little bit." He acknowledged "a couple of other misunderstandings" in which the police had been called but charges were not pressed. Two of these had been with his ex-wives. He related a really pathetic story of a lifetime of broken relationships with business associates, family, friends and his two ex-wives. Taking no responsibility for these failures, he dismissed them with the idea that "people are just no good." As we neared the end of our meeting he started on the topic of some previous visits with other psychiatrists and his angry comments began to get louder and louder. They reached a peak with "those guys were all s.o.b.s and I have a good mind not to come back here".

At this point I said "Al, you can be heard in the waiting room."

He looked at me with a slightly puzzled scowl and shouted, "They can't hear me out there."

I said, "Wait. I'll see." Walking over to the door I opened it, poked my head into the waiting room, and asked "Can you hear us out here?"

My next patient replied, "I can hear some guy in there shouting at the top of his lungs, but I can't hear you."

I said "Thank you. I'll be with you in a few minutes," and closed the door. Al looked somewhat sheepish, and I said, "Al, I've had a number of patients who weren't really aware when they were raising their voice. I think you belong to that group. But because you're not aware that you're doing it you don't realize that it has a disturbing effect on other people and that can be the cause of misunderstandings."

He suddenly asked: "When can I come again?" and I felt like we were off to a good start.

People like Al provoke fights with any professional quite readily, so that they are often treated as though they are less than worthy of our respect. Borderlines are the bane of life for all who dare to hold themselves out as experts on human problems of one kind or another. When they come for help, they often begin with a warning shot about how miserably our colleagues have failed them in the past. They will describe a series of broken relationships with others in any given field, and as they speak of the ineptitude, callousness and preoccupation with money they have encountered, we begin to detect a surge of rage that is headed in our direction. They may well explode in our face with a raw outburst of shocking intensity. It feels like a blast of pure hatred, and that is exactly what it is since it comes from a part of a person that has never been touched by love. It is all the more stunning because its author seems to be a rational person. The urge to counter-punch, or simply walk away (fight or flight) may be quite strong, and yet neither approach would be appropriate or helpful. New York City's late mayor, Fiorello LaGuardia, used to conclude his weekly radio broadcasts in World War II with the words "patience and fortitude." His bit of folksy wisdom in that era when the world was torn by raw aggression should grace the wall above every professional's desk. When we are subjected to a withering attack, we must not flinch under fire. Our calling requires us to accept the bad and worst parts of another with equanimity.

Fortitude is courage based on personal strength and not physical prowess. It is a specifically human quality that allows us to remain calm and hopeful in the face of adversity. Fortitude, a derivative of our inner warmth, operates silently within us to temper our response to those who seek to destroy the bond of good human contact. By focusing on preserving that bond, we can remain unperturbed by our own urges to retaliate. Our inner warmth is then available to meet a hostile attack head-on, and begin the work of getting through.

Patience is part two of the story since the problem, in fact crisis, of these rage explosions, will recur many times. They are part of an automatic interaction that can occur with anyone, especially those in positions of authority. We call these happenings "instant transferences", which means that they are re-enactments of ancient and painful feelings involving parents or siblings. Each time we are subjected to such an attack, it will be experienced as unfair or even a severe injustice. In our certainty that we have done nothing to deserve such an outburst, it is easy to break off the relationship, especially since we may mistakenly assume this is the wish of the client or patient. Fractured relationships are a life-style with them, but not without a price. Every new disruption increases their sense of "badness," because they have driven one more person away from themselves.

When they finally find someone who can accept their hostility without being demolished by it, they experience a profound relief. Soon the attacks become less frequent and less vehement. We begin to realize that we are valued now, perhaps more as a friend than a professional. In the psychotherapeutic relationship a new warmth develops and idealization sets in. We have succeeded in getting through to them and become a valuable part of their life. We can do no wrong for a while until finally anger returns, but in a vastly different form. Gone are the firestorms, reduced to mere temper tantrums that can be studied and resolved, as a result of the sharing of inner warmth.

That is what happened in the case of Al. His hunger for friendship was right out in the open in our second meeting when he began calling me Doctor Jim, and later just Jim. The "getting through" accomplished in our first meeting could be seen in the second when he announced that he needed a new "volume control." Jokes about his faulty "volume control" became one of the major themes of our work, and his ability to laugh at himself served him well. He soon added the need for a new "thermostat" to deal with times when he "got hot under the collar." After a long period in which I could do no wrong he finally "got hot under the collar" with me about one of my comments. After that it became quite easy for him to express his anger at me, but he could also step back and study the reasons why he had become angry.

The need for patience and persistence in working with these individuals is clear. More often than not, we can only accomplish our goals over a long run, since the healing warmth is being directed at long standing maladies. Al's treatment took a little less than five years, thanks to a fortunate marriage. We occasionally run into each other on the street and can always enjoy a good laugh together.

Many psychiatrists have a tendency to distance themselves from working with borderlines. I can trace my own capacity for sharing inner warmth with them directly to my days at Camelot and supervision by Dr. Arnold Modell. He was a man who had a great interest in caring for people who were living with severe overloads of the destructive kind of aggressive energies, and thus became a pioneer in the psychotherapy of both borderlines and schizophrenics. He made himself instantly available for consultation to any of the Fellows who had one of these difficult patients. I have tried to serve my colleagues in the same way.

16

Intimacy, the royal road to personal growth

Intimacy is a special adaptation of inner warmth involving family and friends who share their inner personal warmth along with an expectation of emotional growth on the part of the beneficiary. Julia's treatment was built on the expectation that she could and would come out of her self-centered cocoon and resume her responsibilities as a mother and wife. As we learned at D.C.General, the bond of caring energies that joins us together as a species provides a passageway that is a two-way channel going directly into the interior life of two or more people. The patients at D.C.General were able to help one another escape from profound states of regression by this healing connectedness. The shared inner warmth of intimacy can also be accompanied by an expectation that we will give up infantile behaviors. All of us have our infantile moments that can use some repair. These include impatience, anger, envy, selfishness, seeking control of others, false pride, sexual preoccupations and a tendency to be overly moralistic. Intimacy's mastery over the destructive drives begins at birth and rises to the occasion to modify fresh resurgences of the destructive drives at each new stage of life. The first moments of intimacy occur when a mother and father share their love and bodily warmth with the newborn. Many people have the mistaken notion that babies are born into a blissful existence of sleep and feeding, but their very first emotion is probably rage. After all, they were sleeping soundly in the warm environment of the uterus when they were suddenly awakened by violent muscular contractions. They were squeezed into the narrow confinement of the birth canal with their head or buttocks used as a battering ram. Babies have to be sore all over when they finally emerge into a cold outside world to immediately undergo surgery on the umbilical cord. The first sound they utter is probably a cry of rage. The enormous trauma of the birth process has to create an overload of the destructive drives that brings on the first healing experience in the warm embrace of nurses, mothers and fathers. Soon there are many other sources of pain that give rise to rage and lead to daily experiences of healing. Hunger pains, gastrointestinal colic or muscular cramps intrude upon sleep and awaken the infant in great distress. If a mother is absent or delayed in her response the reaction of rage increases exponentially. The destructive drives that require healing in this era are primitive in nature. We can infer what they are like from those that caused so much terror for Julia in her regressed state. Threatened with desertion by her surrogate mother, (the doctor), she lapsed into urges to tear him into shreds with her teeth or nails, swallow him whole and spit out the pieces. The destructive drive to demolish her doctor also took the form of grinding him into dust on the surface of her skin so that she could blow him away. Both kinds of revenge are characteristic of the rage that has to be healed in the first fifteen months of life. The temper tantrums of the terrible twos use a new weapon, the voluntary musculature, for kicking, hitting and throwing things along with biting and screaming. The urge is simply to destroy by whatever means.

The same people who gave life to their offspring in the uterus provide a secure holding in those first two years. Infants and toddlers are absolutely dependent on the soothing, stroking and loving energies of parents to achieve the modification of their primitive raw aggression.

Repeated experiences in which the fires of infantile rage are extinguished by love create an imprint that sets the life pattern for intimacy. Infants begin as the passive recipients of loving energies from the outside but by the third year they have acquired their own reservoir of loving feelings towards caretakers as part of the "Oedipus complex" described by Freud. A passionate devotion to both parents is evident by then, and love of self begins to give way to love of others. Through intimacy with parents children become active regulators of their loving energies and use them to subdue rage whenever it rears its ugly head. Shame becomes a source of rage at three and four, and wounded gender pride in both sexes increases the intensity of that rage. It is in these years that both parents are taken inside, rules and all, to form the conscience with its set of ideal behavioral guidelines.

The fifth to twelfth years used to be called the latency period, a quiet time for development without undue pressure from the sexual or aggressive drives. It has become a more stormy time with television and movies fanning the fires of sex and violence while the loving instincts are just emerging from infancy. This has made adolescence, when the sexual and aggressive drives do become very strong, a perilous era for a number of individuals who have erupted in homicidal violence towards classmates. The schools have fortunately begun to try to identify troubled students who are at risk for violence and educate their peers in how to take a healing approach towards them. Extremely shy youngsters are often filled with a rage that is the cause of their shyness. Other students are disliked because they bristle with open hostility, and are consequently shunned when, in fact, they need to be healed. The trials and tribulations that have to be mastered in normal adolescence make this a time of major importance in human development. Shared warmth with a teacher, or a few special friends often charts the course of a person's growth for a lifetime.

Romantic love and marriage offer most people their greatest opportunity for the refinement of loving energies through intimacy. This is not just because of the intensity of warmth couples exchange, but even more for the fact that they have to overcome the anger of gender prejudice and wounded gender pride, or the many moments of animosity simply because they are different. Increasingly, in a successful marriage, spouses become loved for how they are, who they are, and how they do differ, rather than how we want them to be. In this way we achieve the maturation of love from its infantile self-centered origins to love of others that are different from ourselves.

Intimacy continues to foster human growth over a lifetime through repeated contests with the destructive drives. Mid-life creates a crisis for quite a few people and a difficult challenge for all. This comes about from the awareness that some of our most cherished wishes for power, wealth or love are not going to be fulfilled. Rage in the form of bitterness confronts many and for some the outcome may be suicide. In mid-life, like adolescence, the destructive drives reach a new level of intensity requiring us to draw on intimacy with family, friends and sometimes counselors to generate ever more powerful and refined loving energies. In our triumph over the rage of the middle years we come out with an enhanced capacity to love that has been called by psychoanalysts a "post-ambivalent" state. Putting aside our preference for abstract terms this means that grandparents can embrace the offspring of their children with a love of superior quality to that given to their own youngsters. It is a love that has less of an admixture with anger or hateful feelings. Grandparents can't always be sweetness and light, however, because they still have to heal the rage that comes from the onslaught of the aging process. The work of intimacy is never done. With each new triumph over the destructive drives our healing potential becomes stronger, preparing us for a peaceful acceptance of death.

Parents, siblings and friends constitute a living, interactive mirror in which we get to know ourselves better, strengthening our conviction about what is good, healthy or admirable in our being, and confronting us, in acceptable ways, with the presence of what is infantile. The "self" is a vital part of the mind, a mental development that begins late in the first year of life as an infant maps out the reaches and functions of its own body and experiences it as separate from a nurturing mother and father. During the next few years, and with steady increments, the "self" develops as a unique agency that monitors the processes of sharing warmth with others, and responding to their encouragement to give up infantile behavior. Gradually, it becomes the "me", the "who I am", a whole range of self-perceptions that are subject to change for the good or bad over the rest of a lifetime.

What is it that shapes the "self," and nourishes good self-esteem? The primary fuel is love, the exchange of inner warmth with family members and later with friends. Good self-esteem also depends on our response to pressure from others to give up infantile behaviors and "grow up." This process begins with parental demands that we control our messy food habits, bowels, bladder, temper tantrums, and other anti-social urges. A great deal of growth can also come about through good-natured banter within a family, and between friends, about our shortcomings.

Freud made us so aware of the crucial impact of those first few years on our later growth that we may tend to overlook the importance of intimate relationships outside the family in determining the kind of person we become. These begin very early. My own childhood offers some good examples. On my very first day at school my mother dropped me off with instructions to come directly home on my own as soon as classes were over. I bonded instantly with the most singular individual in the class—unique because he was the only black youngster. He was also one of the brightest in a typically large parochial school first grade. I invited him home to meet my mom and my aunt. I was proud of my new friend, and regarded our acquaintanceship as the most important accomplishment of my day. I introduced him by his full name, "This is Joseph Grant", and they were duly impressed. Years later I learned that they were also flabbergasted. There were no black children in our neighborhood, and Joe was the first of his race I had ever met.

The next day I visited Joe's home and met his mother and older brother, Julius. I was puzzled at first by his mother, a large black woman who didn't resemble my own mother in any physical way. I asked myself, "How could she be a mom?" I soon had the answer. For she had a great warmth of personality and treated me exactly as she did her own two sons. I was encountering in a relative stranger the same kind of love I knew at home.

Julius was about four years older than Joe, and he became one of my idols. He wore a full-length brace on his right leg, but hobbled nimbly around the apartment. He had inherited much of his mother's warmth, and clearly enjoyed his role as a protector and mentor to his younger brother. Unlike my own big brother, Jack, who was five-years older than I, Julius welcomed the opportunity to play with Joe and me.

Our favorite pastime was football, which we played on the only grassy plot available in the neighborhood, the tiny front yard of a Protestant Church. There was always an air of adventure to our game, since the lot was secured by a wrought iron fence that had to be vaulted to gain access. Once inside we were three Catholic boys in alien Protestant territory, but we used it as our own private park. Two little first-graders and a big fifth-grader, racing across the field, tossing a ball just like the one the New York Giants used. What a boost to our masculine pride. Of course, it took two of us to tackle Julius, but our egos swelled with pride each time we were able to bring down the good natured giant. There were the lessons in humility, too. Often our tackles would turn into wrestling matches, which Julius inevitably won, casting us off like a mighty Houdini as he teased us about our size and strength.

The greater lesson in humility came out of the deep respect we both had for this wonderful big brother who had been able to overcome the handicap left by "infantile paralysis." We marveled at the way he could race across our field, getting an extra spurt of propulsion each time his brace hit the ground. Our respect grew out of the knowledge that his limb was deformed for life and yet he shared a warm and cheerful optimism with us, and wore his brace with pride. My family lived in the Bronx then, and the rich diversity of my closest friends between ages five and nine provided an extraordinary preparation for a later career of working with people who were "different" from myself.

When two or more people begin to exchange inner warmth on a regular basis, the range of feelings that they share may include hopes, fears, embarrassments, sexual feelings, anger, rage, guilt, joy or exhilaration, to name but a few. Just how deeply we can go in this intimacy depends only on the degree of trust we have been able to develop as a result of a steady and reliable exchange of warmth. We depend on other human beings for the abatement of our fears, for confirmation of our sense that we are good people, both loving and lovable, for hope when we edge towards despair, for the acceptance of our anger or even rage when it is justified, or a corrective reappraisal of events when it is not, for relief from the heavy burdens and strictures of a conscience that is too severe and for building a memory bank in which deposits of joy and exhilaration are safely stored, especially the early ones that gather the most interest, so they can be drawn upon in later life when needed.

Those earliest school years with Joe and Julius provided just such an asset in my memory bank, the kind that operates silently and powerfully throughout life. As I mentioned, a majority of the patients at D.C. General were black, and more importantly almost all of the male and female nursing assistants were black. The simpatico I felt with the staff was extraordinary, and it allowed us to have the freest informal discussions about patients I have ever known. There was no holding back, on their part or mine. We felt able to say everything we thought or felt about those we were trying to help. We respected and learned from each other, and consequently our knowledge about patients was greatly strengthened, and care plans were carried out with conviction. In theory, these were teaching sessions for the nursing staff. In reality they were refreshingly intimate experiences of learning for all of us. I have no doubt where my ease of communication and sense of team harmony came from. Even without conscious awareness on my part, it was the replication of the same joyful behavior pattern that I remembered from the days with Joe and Julius.

About 30 years after the unlocking of D.C. General, I was walking through the crowded lobby of the Washington Hospital Center when I heard my name being called out from the far side of the room. "Dr. Ryan, Dr. Ryan." I couldn't see who was calling me until, suddenly, the figure of an elderly man emerged from the milling crowd. He was weaving his way across the lobby, hurrying, as he hobbled along with a cane. Shades of Julius. It was George Gibbs, a nursing assistant from D.C.General.

We spent 20 minutes in happy reunion sharing memories in great detail. He still couldn't believe the changes we had seen in our work, and he thanked me over and over again for what he said were the best years of his life. His gratitude was no greater than my own towards him, which was deeply heartfelt. That shared memory and brief interval of intimacy made my day, week and month. It renewed my belief in the importance of those earliest experiences of intimacy.

Before my days at D.C. General the greatest professional growth I had known occurred during two years as a fellow in psychiatry at the Beth Israel Hospital in Boston. On a visit home after about two months at the B.I., I was telling my parents about what a marvelous training center it was. My father wondered if I found it much different working with mostly Jewish doctors and patients, after my years at the Georgetown University Hospital where the majority of doctors, and patients as well, were Catholic. I thought about it and said, "You know, that's a very good question. I had my greatest year of training as an intern in internal medicine at Georgetown, and then enjoyed two years there in neurology and psychiatry. I had a lot of good friends all around the hospital, and in fact I was the Social Chairman of the House Staff for three years. I thought it was going to be very hard to leave a place I liked so much, but I felt right at home at Beth Israel almost from the very beginning. I just seemed to fit right in. It's my kind of hospital. I'd have to say I like it better than Georgetown. Yes, it's my new home."

My father reminded me, "Maybe that's because you grew up in the Bronx." And then he added, "You know when we lived there, your brother Jack's friends were all from St. John's School, but you used to play with the Jewish kids on our street every day. You even asked if you couldn't go to religion classes at the Synagogue with them."

My comfort level at the B.I. was no genetic accident, but more likely a product of the memory bank of happy early intimacy. It set the stage for a career as a Freudian psychoanalyst that began when I took the advice of my mentors at Beth Israel and entered the "orthodox" Baltimore Psychoanalytic Institute for seven more years of post-graduate training in a predominantly Jewish specialty.

I emphasize the richness of sources of intimacy other than family and spouse, because there are so many who do not have spouses or families available in their lives. If that is the case there's no need for despair because the shortfall of emotional fuel from these traditional resources can be compensated for by many other kinds of intimate human experience. Membership in church or alumni groups, clubs like my favorite University Club in Washington, charitable groups, book clubs, hiking clubs, or any kind of hobby club, all offer a wonderful springboard for making new friends, or even sharing warmth with strangers.

Intimacy is a Gulf Stream that flows through our lives, bringing inner warmth from person to person, spreading it out among others, nourishing their minds and bodies with it, carrying a message to do their best from one to another and uniting all who are touched by this bountiful stream. It speaks once again to a purposefulness in human existence for the good of each other, for a sharing that goes beyond inner warmth, and involves the exchange of knowledge about our weaknesses, and needs for improvement.

Intimacy can even reach out from the grave, and powerfully take hold of those who have been emotionally close to the deceased, as I learned at the funeral of my friend, Dr. John Kuhn. John was a suburban physician who did some volunteer work in Washington. He was about 15 years older than I, and I really only got to know him well in the last three years of his life. He was retired by that time but still played a larger-than-life role in the existence of the many who had benefited from his care. He was to my way of thinking the perfect doctor, a dedicated obstetrician who knew what it was to work a 24-hour day. Hippocrates must have had such a man in mind when he set out the highest standards for our profession. John was also a very humble person.

I once asked him what he did as a volunteer because I had briefly considered working at the same place, which was a residence for homeless men, and hospice for people critically ill with AIDS. I knew that he went there one afternoon a week with his good friend Shep Abell, a very caring lawyer. "I'm just Shep's gopher," was his reply. Together they were spending their time with the men in the AIDS hospice, as companions, and indeed as gophers for those who were immobilized by illness.

"Gift of Peace" was the name of this center for human care, and it was run by nuns from the Order of Mother Teresa. When I had gone there as a potential volunteer it was with the idea that I might be able to offer some kind of psychiatric help with medication or psychotherapy. On a tour through the building it was obvious that there was no need for my professional services. The homeless men seemed quite content even without access to television, and the AIDS patients were resting most of the time, and awaiting their death with equanimity.

I asked Sister Manorama how many had died within the past year and she produced a list from her pocket with the names of the 18 men who had succumbed over the previous two years. She was keeping it to help her remember them in her prayers. A number of her colleagues could be heard at prayer in the chapel, and the whole building seemed to be alive with white robed angels of mercy busy with many tasks, including wiping down the walls with an antiseptic agent. I was very impressed with how much was being accomplished there, but left without any immediate plan to come back, unsure that I could be of help.

John passed away about three years later. His funeral was a very moving experience for me, evoking a real sense of loss at the death of such a good man. I kept thinking of our conversation about his role at "Gift of Peace." Here was this great physician telling me that he was only a gopher, and yet he clearly felt that his efforts were worthwhile, and he was full of admiration and gratitude for Shep who had introduced him to this work.

As we followed his casket from the church, I had an unexpected idea: "I'm going to go to 'Gift of Peace', Shep will need a new helper". John and I had not been "close friends," but we were "good friends" who had gotten to know each other's thinking about healing quite well, and enjoyed comparing notes about our work as doctors. He had helped to strengthen my conviction about what I was writing. His gopher self-description had returned to haunt my soul, and become a part of me. John's humility stood in marked contrast to the pride that had blinded me to the real needs of the men at "Gift of Peace" on my first visit there. He was guiding me now to a place of great beauty and under-standing where there would be an opportunity to heal my pride.

Pride is a funny thing, a simple word that has so many different shades of meaning. We speak of ourselves as being justly proud when we have done something well for which we know that we deserve credit. I realized that I had allowed pride in my professional attainment to dis-tract me from the courage of those who were struggling to survive a debilitating disease, and to maintain human dignity in an illness stig-matized by society. These were people who really needed the deep per-sonal support, and strengthening of faith and hope that can only come from a healing intimate relationship. I soon learned at "Gift of Peace" what a joyful intimacy it was possible to have with the dying, the physi-cally handicapped, or the homeless who were profoundly down on their luck. I saw men fight to stay alive, and then face death without com-plaint and even with serenity, knowing that they possessed within the love of those around them. The fight was fierce, but the final hours were peaceful. It's easy to have the delusion that we are better than oth-ers, but it dissolves fast when you have intimate friends like the men at "Gift of Peace." Life gets more relaxed when you can tone down your self-assessment and accept your equal footing with others.

17

The healing physician, an endangered species

There is a rich intimacy in the doctor-patient relationship that plays a powerful role in the healing of medical illness. The physician's personal warmth and careful listening can be more important than the medication that is finally prescribed. Some patients feel better just being in the presence of a caring doctor. They can vent their anger, express their frustrations with jobs or marriages, reveal very private bodily fears, and know their secrets are safely kept and humanely understood. When illnesses are serious and life threatening, or include prolonged physical suffering, they generate unconscious rage, which can be modified by the doctor's care and concern. The exchange of inner warmth in such circumstances is as vital to survival as the "warming point" was to the well being of schizophrenics.

A coalition of social scientists, technicians, and businessmen are determined to substitute their own perception of what is helpful for the sick to replace the care, concern, ability and judgment of the old-fashioned, healing physician. They operate most commonly under the collective name of "Managed Care." To paraphrase Cicero, it is time for the medical profession to cry out in one loud voice: "How long, O Managed Care, will you continue to try our patience?" (And abuse our patients). "O tempora, O mores." Managed Care, now there is one of the great oxymorons of all time. Think about it. Can these two words really fit together? Can you squeeze just the right amount of care from a tube?

Care comes from the heart, and is the most precious gift a doctor has to give. A young doctor has to own a certain amount of it to begin with, because it is going to be the driving force behind all he or she does thereafter. A doctor has to learn an awful lot about people, more than he ever dreamed would be possible, in order to help them. Only love for people, and love for his profession, will enable him to do this happily. If a doctor's motive is greed, he or she will likely depart the medical vineyard prematurely and always be an outsider to colleagues. If the motive is love, new discoveries about patients will attend a doctor's efforts, and growth in scientific knowledge as well. What a tragedy for mankind, if care is to be sacrificed to the interests of more efficient management.

I am afraid that Managed Care would mandate the denial of coverage for most of the healing approaches discussed in this book. Even Dr. Harvey might have been in trouble had they known he was admitting a terminal case just to let a family know that everything possible had been done. The fact that his bedside presence at the moment of death was an enormous consolation to the bereaved would count for little in today's medical marketplace. Dr. Bibring's sometimes life-saving consultations for uncooperative patients might be barred by contractual stipulations that exclude the treatment-resistant individual. As for psychiatrists trying to augment medication through artful psychotherapy that is no longer available even in the highest option plan.

The irony in this assault on the medical ideal of the caring physician is that the health care planners have sacrificed the surest way in which to control medical costs. Those who care the most about it could best reform a profession that has been based on love since the time of Hippocrates. Most doctors do worry about the burdensome costs that patients must bear, and they know better than anyone else what can be done to reduce them.

During my medical internship at Georgetown University Hospital we had a weekly "Death Conference" to examine in minute detail the treatment of every patient who had just expired. The medical sub-specialists and pathologists who participated in these reviews with the house staff were totally candid in their appraisal of what had been good or bad about our work. But the star-performer in these meetings was almost invariably one of the medical residents, Dr. John Tuohy.

Dr. Tuohy had an encyclopedic knowledge of the cost of every drug, brand and generic, and every lab test or diagnostic procedure recorded in the chart. He came armed with a pocket calculator in order to show the doctor-generated cost of treatment, and then would discuss alternate diagnostic and therapeutic strategies that often might have saved several thousand dollars. The man was a genius in medical economics and left us with much to ponder about how we were managing our cases. When the White House assembled its panel of experts to meet in secret on Universal Health Care, were there any Dr. Tuohys at the table?

It seems to me that the most rational way to formulate a plan for Universal Health Care would have been to gather a group of treating and caring physicians in each state to exploit both the goodness of their hearts and their expertise at cost reduction. The academics and big money winners from successful specialty groups would not have been needed in the room, although their thinking on every subject would have been appropriate for the treating doctors to consider. Our tradition of cutting costs goes back to Hippocrates, and care, which is the primary determinant of our work, antedates him. I truly believe that if a few good physicians in each state had been given the current costs of treatment, along with a dollar figure for the savings needed to produce Universal Health Care, it would exist today.

Some of the most promising initiatives for reducing the costs of medical care have already received the strong encouragement of doctors. Physicians are well aware that they have no monopoly on the power to heal. The potential of human beings to provide healing experiences to one another has been in focus throughout this book, and physicians have a rich tradition of using every possible source of auxiliary help for their patients. As a result, the use of support groups to combat almost every conceivable type of chronic or life-threatening illness has been dramatically on the rise throughout the country. Typically, these groups allow people suffering from the same malady to share intimate details about their hardships and coping mechanisms.

Every serious illness is accompanied by arousal of the aggressive drives, including some elements of the destructive drives. When the very existence of our "self" is threatened, the instinct to fight gets stirred up. The fact that the body itself has ceased to function in its usual way is also a constant source of self-centered torment, and indignation. To cope with this sudden surplus of the destructive drives, family and friends rally around the sick person with a fresh supply of love. Most of us can also use some help from the outside. Human beings who are faced with the same disaster are uniquely positioned to help one another, and in the process, they experience a double gain. By extending their care and concern to others, they increase the supply of loving energies available within themselves for their own needs.

There are other psychological advantages to such support groups. They strengthen people's identity as sufferers from a particular illness, increasing their acceptance of the condition. At the same time, they provide some outward discharge of the destructive drives by way of aggressive campaigns for more research or better treatment. The record of the various support groups' success rate is still a matter for further study, but I think it's safe to predict they will out-perform traditional medical and surgical approaches that do not include group support.

Collaboration between the medical profession and Church groups has already lowered the costs of care in the mental health field. The Anchor Mental Health Program in Washington is a good example of one such medical-religious alliance worthy of imitation in other cities. It all began 40 years ago when St. Elizabeth's Hospital was still the home to seven thousand long-term residents, and only a few would trickle out onto the streets of Washington each week. A number of these people took comfort in attending Mass at St. Matthew's Cathedral in downtown D.C., where they met up with a young priest just out of the seminary who had a bright idea. Fr. John Kuhn started a club for them, calling it the "Anchor Club" to designate its hopeful, stabilizing purpose. It met on weekends for a community supper.

He soon recognized that many of these chronic schizophrenics had trouble finding a place to live and so the first Anchor House was started, with a live-in counselor for added support. In time other Anchor Houses and apartments were established, and the Anchor Club became a daily operation. A large warehouse was acquired to house a training program in janitorial work, and food service. It also had income from government mailing contracts, and salaried jobs for the trainees. Finally a hands-on casework program was established with a staff who knew how to find the mentally ill in their favorite haunts, and set up meetings on park benches or street corners when necessary. They would meet their clients while still in the hospital and literally walk them out into the community, teaching them how to manage their finances and travel the city on public transportation.

Almost all of their clients are on lifetime regimens of anti-psychotic medication, but in spite of this, a good many lapse into psychosis that once would have catapulted them back into the hospital. The Anchor personnel know how to get through to them during these episodes of withdrawal, delusions and hallucinations. As a result, over 95% of their referrals have been able to remain out of the hospital and most of these eventually become self-supporting.

Anchor is now the second largest supplier of mental health care in Washington outranked only by St. Elizabeth's. It has recently entered the arena of care for the homeless with a contract to provide treatment for 100 known psychotics who are living on the streets. Most of these people have developed serious addictions to drugs or alcohol as part of their desperate efforts to dampen rage and quiet inner turmoil. They require even greater degrees of supervision and supportive staff interaction than patients coming directly from the hospital, but the early results are encouraging. Here again, the patience and persistence of caretakers are vital to their recovery. Already 55 out of the first 64 referrals have been established in permanent housing and gotten started on productive lives.

The Anchor program holds great promise for the development of more effective treatment for both acute and chronic mental illness, as well as the addictions, with a vast saving in cost. It is well supervised as to quality of care, with a good scattering on staff of people who hold master's degrees. However, most of its caretakers begin with college-level education, and they acquire their expertise in mental health while on the job. What matters is their dedication and personal warmth, and they are carefully selected with these characteristics in mind.

In order to arrive at an effective program of Universal Health Care the public mental health clinics are going to have to work closely with organizations such as Anchor. This has already happened in Washington where Anchor acts as an extension of the clinics, monitoring the use of medication and quickly reporting on problems. The many church groups actively serving the homeless could also act as auxiliaries of the clinics. Their loyal and caring volunteers could provide the kind of warmth needed by schizophrenics and drug users as well.

18

Overcoming prejudice

Looking back on the healing of schizophrenics at D.C.General I'm unsure as to the most important accomplishment of our staff. Certainly they provided a wealth of new information about our human nature but I think they achieved something much more notable. They were able to overcome one of the oldest and most powerful prejudices in humankind, contempt for the mentally ill. Prejudice puts a lock on human progress, especially in our social exchanges with other people, and also on the growth of our knowledge about them. The staff at D.C.General not only unlocked all its doors, but they also opened a gaping hole in a wall of prejudice that was holding schizophrenics hostage, condemning them to abuse and shielding them from scientific inquiry.

When we are faced with the unwanted chore of getting through to those we dislike, most of us probably think: "Why would I want to get through to someone I despise? I stay as far away from those kind of people as I can." The answer is a simple one. It may be one of the best things you can do for your health.

"Those kind of people" might be members of a different race, creed, national background, social status or political party. The speaker could be you or I, and we might well be "those kind of people" to someone else. Prejudice is so ubiquitous that we take it to be an ordinary part of human nature. Often it is so much a part of who we are that we feel quite comfortable with it and wouldn't think of trying to make a change. So what's the big deal?

Well, actually it can be a very big deal. Prejudice is the hiding place for destructive drives. We take a portion of this dark underside of our make-up, and adorn it with enough rationalizations to create a wolf in sheep's clothing. Thus removed from any contact with our inner warmth, these hostile feelings are kept at bay, but they retain their raw instinctual, predatory potential. In other words, we have made a commitment to this segment of our destructive drives that they will remain unmodified.

We are born with destructive drives, but they are substantially altered by parental love. Still, as we know too well, the human animal can kill if necessary, and often when it's not necessary. When we have had an experience that enrages us the urge to kill is aroused and sleep becomes more difficult. The presence of the destructive drives in everyone is the single greatest source of anxiety, panic and insomnia.

The subjugation of these drives is an ongoing task throughout life since different ages produce new stimuli for rage. To the extent that we are successful in this endeavor, we heal ourselves, and advance the cause of our health both emotionally and physically. Healing occurs whenever we are able to allow our inner warmth to blend with our destructive urges. Without healing, anger becomes rationalized, and pride is buoyed by the false notion that we are better in one way or another than some of our fellow human beings. Our knowledge of reality is consequently impaired, and we remain ever vulnerable to anxiety.

In any kind of prejudice we draw a sharp line between a class of people whom we believe to be wrong, even evil, and the rest of us who are good, or better or best. Such a cleavage has a clear stamp of the infantile. It brings to mind the well known nursery rhyme: "There was a little girl, And she had a little curl, Right in the middle of her forehead,

And when she was good, she was very, very good, And when she was bad, she was horrid." It was probably written about a two-year-old, and needless to say, it has equal validity for a boy of that age. Before the second year, children also tend to experience their parents as either all-good or all-bad, and only gradually come to recognize that it is one and the same mother or father who can be both loved and hated. And so their behavior fluctuates between exquisite tenderness, and those terrible tantrums in which their hateful outbursts have not yet been modified by their love.

A simple prejudice diverts some of our hateful feelings away from those we hold dear, by shunting our anger towards an outside group. The late Dr. David Rappaport was a brilliant scholar of psychoanalysis who used humor to good effect on the topic of how even people of the same religion may deal with the admixture of love and hate towards one another. He told the following joke at grand rounds in Boston's Beth Israel hospital: "During World War II, there was a Jewish sailor who had the misfortune of being washed from the deck of his ship in a sudden squall. He clung to a piece of driftwood as his ship steamed on into the night, and by the next day he landed on a remote South Pacific isle. He quickly befriended the natives who were ready to grant his every wish, and accordingly he asked them to build a temple. When it was completed he asked them to build a second one, which they did without question. After many months, a U.S. Naval vessel appeared offshore, and their crew responded to his signals by sending a rescue launch. The captain was astonished when he saw the first edifice on the island, but he was utterly incredulous to find a second. He said that he thought it had been a wonderful idea to have a temple in which the castaway might pray for his deliverance, but why the second one? Whereupon the sailor replied, "Well Sir, it's very simple. The first temple is the one in which I worship; but as for the second, that one, I wouldn't be seen dead in it."

The anecdote neatly illustrates the absurdity of our prejudice, and also holds out the possibility that we may be able to overcome this rational flaw by learning to laugh at ourselves. The maxim that warns us not to engage in the discussion of religion or politics at social gatherings has a very sound basis in developmental psychology. We tend to adorn our religious and political beliefs with a precious mantle of certitude for which we are ready to fight at a moment's notice. When our destructive energies are placed in the service of "all-good" causes, they may even lead to terrible persecutions and "Holy Wars", as in our present world crisis.

Like it or not, we have a cruel streak in our nature that can only be modified when we admit love to the mix. That is not only the foremost task of our childhood development but also the greatest challenge of our mature years. When we succeed in overcoming a prejudice, we tone down our more primitive and eruptive hostile drives and emerge with a greater sense of security. We become less afraid of ourselves and of others as well. By reducing our "stranger anxiety," we'll find that we can learn a great deal from others who are different.

Schizophrenics are about as different as any one class of human beings can be from the rest of us. Centuries of ignorance about the nature of their illness permitted their execution as witches, or as creatures possessed by the devil. Finally in 1786, Phillipe Pinel took the bold step of releasing them from their chains in the Salpetriere in Paris, and returning them to society. Almost two centuries later they were again in exile by the tens of thousands in huge state hospitals, while the parade of modern medicine passed them by.

We were taught in the early 50's that some of these patients might recover if it was their first episode of illness, and a few might even survive their first recurrence. But a third hospitalization had an aura of doom, and the certain prognosis of a lifetime of incarceration in the state hospital. We didn't understand that each of these patients was also possessed of a perfectly rational mind that needed only good human contact with another person to gain the strength to function, and reassert its dominance over their craziness. Albeit they sometimes had to go through recurrences that were now short-lived.

Why did it take us so long to find out this simple truth? The answer in two words is human prejudice, one of the oldest and most deeply entrenched in mankind. In the acute stages of their illness schizophrenics are so very different that it is easy to conveniently assign almost any trait, tendency, fear, flaw or even potential weakness that we disliked in ourselves to them. Having thus disposed of our imperfections, it was only natural to banish these carriers of our faults from polite society.

Schizophrenics' illnesses had begun with the deepest possible kind of withdrawal from personal involvement with others. Without good human contact, the mental processes of these patients became subject to a wide range of aberrations. But their treatment in the 1950's, and in many places still today, consisted chiefly in segregation, even from their families and friends, so that the damage from the initial wound of withdrawal was enormously compounded. Often their behavior within the walls of the state hospital was much more disturbed than it had been without. If you had had occasion to visit one of these "warehouses of the mentally ill," you would have seen an open display of all of man's worst fears about himself within a very short time. The diversity and intensity of these basic fears provided a rich soil for the tenacious roots of prejudice.

A look at hospital life in the fifties would have said it all about why we needed to create such distance between these patients and ourselves. First, there was the chaos and apparent loss of control over rational thought. The fear of going crazy is one of those universal human worries, present in all of us at one time or another. It is especially strong in adolescence when powerful new sexual and aggressive drives strain the containment capacities of a still childish ego. Many have already had their parents admonish them not to touch their "private parts" lest they become insane and have to be "put away." But even those who have not heard this ridiculous warning make a ready connection between the outlet of masturbation and the danger that this activity may allow their sexual drives to come cascading through with overpowering force.

In the bygone era of sexual explanations for all the vagaries of human conduct, we might have stopped here in our endeavor to explain the pervasiveness of prejudice towards the mentally ill. In the process we would have been relieved of the burden of confronting the much more disturbing anxieties that attend our hostile drives. Our patients in that era were surely the living occupants of Hell consumed by their own internal conflagration, and damned by society for their sins of wanton sexuality and uncontrolled violence. Their withdrawal served to protect the rest of us from danger, but it robbed them of the comfort of warm and secure feelings. They were unloving and unlovable, empty, cold, hollow shells of humanity. With so much reality to support a prejudice of centuries, it seems remarkable to me that the staff at D.C. General Hospital was able to go so far in overcoming their own prejudice.

Thorazine, the first of the major tranquilizing drugs, had been in use during that time, and even at St. Elizabeth's the noise level had come down. The drug was capable of transforming unrestrained violence into sleep, and seemed to take the edge off of delusions, although their content remained the same. The recovery rate for schizophrenics hadn't changed at D.C. General, but staff morale received a lift from Thorazine. This provided a starting point for their eventual triumph over prejudice, for now everyone, patients and staff, had some hope.

Hope is the wellspring of human initiative. Without it a patient has no reason to struggle to overcome any illness, and death seems a release. The anticipation that things can get better is what we live for. With our own short supply of this vital therapeutic ingredient, we on the staff had almost none to offer our patients. Ultimately we came to realize that the clear expectation of staff that patients could and would control their behavior was crucial to the patients' recovery of self-control.

Our nursing staff was mostly black, and those who dealt with the violent were mostly male. What manner of men were these, who could take a spark of hope and generate a bountiful confidence in themselves so they might give a boost to others? They were family men, with a deeply rooted spirituality nurtured through generations of oppression. They understood the unique personal value of each and every human as a child of God, and related to patients accordingly. They were more than ready to expect the best of patients, and willing to take the risk of extending their inner warmth to many, who were likely to reject the offer. They were able to rise above the ordinary; to go beyond what was normally expected of human behavior, and achieve the accomplishments I've described. They were the four minute milers of psychiatry. How different from the familiar stereotype of our prejudice.

The women staffers had been born into the same rich spiritual tradition, so that they too were well prepared to do more, be more, and go beyond. They were equally courageous and hopeful when confronting the open hostility, potential violence or severe withdrawal of our patients. It was precisely in this way that our staff made its greatest leap. For the instinctual forces that were driving patient behaviors were of the most primitive and destructive variety, and could easily evoke a response in kind from the caretakers. (An eye for an eye, and a tooth for a tooth.)

The human fight or flight apparatus is exquisitely sensitive to the type of drive pressures exhibited by schizophrenics. To say it in another way, the gut response centers of our staff were under constant bombardment. Their own urges to fight were being mobilized countless times each day by hostility from patients, but they successfully quieted these urges by blending them with their deep concern for others. They were thus able to accept the hostile and crazy otherness of their patients and relate to them with warmth rather than fear.

The warming point in schizophrenia described in Chapter Five represented the patients' response to the unusual care and hope provided by the staff. It marked the return of their own capacity to permit the intermingling of their loving and hateful feelings. The split between the psychotic and the non-psychotic selves had at least been bridged, and the healing process was under way. The ability of our staff to relate to patients as whole people, and accept their badness along with their goodness helped patients to become less afraid of their own hostility, so that they could resume the basic human task of using their love to modify and overcome their hatred.

An important lesson for all of us in this account of one group's triumph over prejudice is the personal growth and improved ability to love that came from this experience. Shortly after the great unlocking, our Chief Psychologist, the genial Dr. Bernie Levy, came bursting into my office with an important discovery. "I've just come from the George Washington University Hospital (where he was also the Chief of Psychology) and I can't get over the difference between the staffs there and here. They're tired, depressed and irritable, while over here everyone looks rested, energetic and friendly." I valued Bernie's comments, as he was a very perceptive man, and began to make observations of my own during the next month in the two private hospitals where I had staff privileges. My findings were just the same as his. It was really hard to believe that these other groups were engaged in the same occupation as our staff.

It is possible, of course, that our personnel were more well rested, but we have already discussed how the quality of sleep is often a measure of one's command over their own aggressive drives. Fitful rest is the natural outcome of a day's residue of destructive urges. Our staff had conquered and subdued their anger with love, and probably were blessed with better sleep. Certainly, their greater self-content by day was undeniable.

Do you want to be less afraid? Find yourself a group of people who are neglected by others, and get involved in regular visits with them as a volunteer. Schizophrenics in a half-way house will do, or prisoners in a jail. Then there are the far-advanced elderly in nursing homes that have few visitors, and the terminally ill with AIDS or cancer. You will find yourself with a new set of friends possessed of a precious inner warmth that has survived in the face of adversity. Your interest will help to fuel this warmth, which in turn will rekindle your own sense of how special it is to be human. And you will see, convincingly, how the forces of love remain dominant over our rage even unto the end.

When you can invest in people who are quite different from yourself, you will be able to develop and enhance your ability to love, for you will experience the most maturing, and mature kind of love, a love that embraces the otherness and individuality of someone you care for.

19

Volunteer activities to heal our infantile self

Psychoanalysts have their infantile behaviors just like everyone else. With four or five hours a week of training analysis we probably absorb more therapy than any other group of people. The sad fact is that analysts have almost as many marital failures, and parental shortcomings, as the rest of the population. We can lose our temper, be impatient, envy others, know it all, and engage in power struggles with the best. Our lengthy and thorough analyses are unquestionably strengthening, but the infantile core of the self must still be dealt with over a lifetime.

What makes the infantile core so resistant to change? In earliest childhood there is a substantial disparity between the strengths of the infant's own loving and destructive instincts. The love drives are still highly self-centered, and dependent on loving in-put from a mother and father, at a time when the destructive drives are being unleashed on the outside world in full force. The love experiences are intimately linked with pleasurable feelings, and there is a tendency to hold on to the love/pleasure feelings for as long as possible to soothe the self, and thereby protect it from the arousal of the destructive drives. Clinging to love and pleasure feelings is further guarded by the process of splitting in which loving and hateful feelings, and their targets, are carefully segregated into all-good and all-bad categories of experience. Splitting tends to preserve the hateful urges in their most destructive infantile form, leaving them much stronger than the loving instincts that are constantly in need of refueling from the outside. This fateful split leaves us forever afraid that our destructive urges may overcome and annihilate the loving core of our makeup. We are left with the lifelong task of modifying the destructive drives in order to reassure ourselves that the urge to destroy remains under our dominance. If we succeed in further subjugating our raw aggression, it will become less necessary to hold on to infantile behaviors, and our maturing self will be freer to use aggressive energies for productive purposes.

How can we best modify the infantile core of our makeup? The various schools of psychotherapy, including psychoanalysis, each have their own helpful approaches to problem solving but we are still left with the infantile core of our make-up. Psychotherapy is based on an appeal to the rational side of man's nature, i.e. to a strengthening of the ego. Unfortunately the problem is deeply rooted in the id, the powerful destructive drives of man, the animal, that force him to keep the id at bay without actually changing it.

Inner warmth, our greatest therapeutic resource, must be given direct access to the id so that it can tone down the destructive drives. That can only be done through action, and life experience, and not by reasoning. There are two ways in which we can engage the id with the healing love of inner warmth. The first way has to do with directly reducing the impact of our own id on relationships with family, friends and other people generally. The second is to be of help to others who are struggling with an overload of the destructive energies in their id.

The problem with the first approach is that the id tends to be a sneaky customer. Remember prejudice, the wolf in sheep's clothing? Male chauvinists and women's libbers are not the only ones who deal in gender prejudice. Men and women are so different physically and emotionally that gender issues have to be confronted in every marriage. The id impulses that lurk behind this prejudice can produce very sharp words that seriously wound gender pride, especially in the early years of a marriage. If the wounds are not treated immediately through the restoration of good human contact, they become grudges that live on for a lifetime. How best to improve a marriage? Work on the grudges with the goal of arriving at forgiveness. What a waste of emotional energy that they reappear year after year or month after month. They represent a part of the id that's still a loose cannon on the deck.

It isn't really the id that tends to be sneaky, it is a wily part of the ego that rationalizes about that old insult to pride and tells us we have good reason to hold on to the grudge. The real reason for its persistence is the memory of the power of that long ago rage reaction and the wish to avoid its reactivation. The grudge represents a compromise with the id. The person who can reach out to heal an old wound to pride in any relationship achieves a final victory over an old upsurge of his or her id.

A lesser degree of vengefulness often divides siblings who have drifted apart. Their problems may have begun early in life around a competition about who is the favorite of mom or dad. Another sore spot can be who was given more, or in the present, who has more. Many grow apart because of differing lifestyles. "We just don't have much in common anymore" is often the byword of siblings who have only telephone contact at yearly intervals, if that. They miss out on the special kind of shared warmth that comes from early life togetherness, and can be powerfully healing even over the telephone. Visits with siblings several times a year, and contact by telephone at regular intervals and on holidays helps to keep the glow of family love alive. Sibling love is the vintage kind. It draws on parental love, grows and matures over the years, and does wonders for an overload of destructive energies. A long separation can be followed by a reunion that will restore regular contact. Happy the person who makes the first move in that direction. And happy, too, is the recipient.

There is a simple, every day, exercise that can bring our healing love into contact with residues of the destructive drives. Stranger anxiety is another "normal" prejudice, even more acceptable to most of us than gender prejudice. Walking down the street we're liable to smile and say good morning or hello to a stranger who is dressed like we are. Clothe that man or woman in a different attire, or foreign garb, and we're more likely to pass them by without greeting. If they appear to be homeless we may move away, and more quickly. Why not a warm and friendly good morning for everyone? If they respond in kind both of us will feel better for it. If not, at least we know that we have shown our respect for a fellow human being. The fear that we may get a hostile response is based on our own hostility towards someone we fear may be harmful. To reach a warming point with such a person helps to tame our basic hostility and mistrust of strangers.

The other way of modifying the id is by offering hands-on care to people who are outcasts of society. Their number includes persons whose bodies have been ravaged by diseases like cancer and AIDS. To serve them as a volunteer places you instantly in alien human territory. Your basic sense that it is only right and fair for the human body to remain intact is going to be assaulted by sights, sounds and smells that evoke revulsion. We have a "normal" human prejudice warning us to keep away from people like that.

As with any prejudice our own rage is just around the corner, signaling us not to put it to the test. In earlier Freudian days we might have said that we avoid those who are physically debilitated and dying because of our anxiety about bodily damage. This prejudice has much deeper roots than that, taking us into the raw aggression of the most primitive portion of the mind. After all we're talking here about people who are living prematurely on death's row, and must be suffused with unconscious rage in addition to an oversupply of conscious rage. They are also being subjected to the serial destruction of vital bodily functions. In such circumstances, the "seething cauldron" of the id is boiling over.

Volunteers who spend a few hours each week with the seriously ill or dying participate very intimately in their struggle with raw instinctual energies. They become strongly identified with the group, so that their own id gets exposed to healing warmth as they share warmth with those whom they serve.

The taming of the id can also be achieved by more frequent visits with friends who are desperately ill. We let friends slowly slip away, knowing they are doing so and "thinking" of visiting, and suddenly it is too late. The basic reason for this missed opportunity is fear of our own destructive drives. Death is the ultimate weapon of the id. We may secretly wish it for others, but only rarely and briefly for ourselves. To visit with the dying requires the contemplation of our own final destruction, and the consequent quickening of rage within the id. Add to this our resonance with what we sense must be going on inside a friend, and it becomes easier to stay away. It is indeed a missed opportunity for both the victim of illness, and our personal growth.

"I'd like to go see poor Bill, but he looked terrible the last time I ran into him, and I just don't know what we could talk about. Anything I say about what we've been doing lately is going to make him feel bad (envious). It isn't just about golf or restaurants, but even taking walks. And it's just so difficult for me to look at him." It is hard to look at someone who is wasting away, but the best kind of looking is eye-to-eye in order to express the full depth of one's compassion. Even as with mother and infant, it is the most direct channel for the conveyance of a deep respect and affection. It transcends the distressing sight and heals the related emotional wounds.

Words aren't important, except for "Hello Bill", but handholding is, and maybe some stroking with the other hand. The bed-ridden will often supply the words, describing their day-to-day experiences in touchingly minute detail. You may have approached the visit with trepidation, and ended it with a sadness that is held within, but you will depart with the sure knowledge that both visitor and patient are better for it.

We've been talking about some pretty tough assignments for the exercise of healing love. Jails and subway grates, AIDS and cancer wards, halfway houses for the mentally ill or addicted, are not exactly exciting places in which to hang out. But they are rich in opportunity for encounters with the id. Healing love becomes activated in a unique way, and provides an emergency transfusion of hope to people overwhelmed by rage and despair. An active love with outreach to others quite different from ourselves increases within us, and strengthens confidence in the mastery of our own id impulses. The quality of sleep is improved, other love relationships become more secure, and vulnerability to anxiety is reduced.

Most of us have some degree of aversion to the environments just mentioned. I'd like to add one more to the list; one that might be more appealing, and yet it has received even less volunteer attention than any of the places above. I'm referring to the homes for the far-advanced elderly, most of who require considerable nursing care.

A few years ago I was asked if I could provide consultation at one such place, to monitor overly aggressive patients and regulate their dosage with the medication Haldol, a heavy-duty tranquilizer. I had never been to the facility, though it housed over 200 people, had a good reputation, and had been the final home for the parents of several of my patients.

I was frankly reluctant to go, rationalizing my resistance on the basis of the one-hour round-trip, a busy practice, and my limited experience with people in their late eighties and nineties. These patients all were suffering from either Senile or Arteriosclerotic Dementia, or Alzheimer's Disease. What I really had was a bad case of stranger-anxiety as well as the mistaken assumption that little could be done for someone with dementia. I remember telling myself, "You felt the same way about schizophrenia when you were younger," and that finally tipped the scale in favor of the trip.

I arrived at the venerable institution on a brilliant fall afternoon. The handsome brick structure sat atop a knoll graced with blazing autumnal foliage, providing a postcard picture image of the perfect retirement home. An elderly woman in her Sunday best chatted out front with a young visitor to complete the tranquil scene.

Inside, the marble lobby created some foreboding since its chairs were unoccupied by either residents or visitors. I made my solitary way by a creaky elevator to the third floor where the door opened upon a ghastly scene. There were about eight wheelchairs arranged in a circle, each containing a very aged human being who looked almost moribund. They neither talked with, nor looked at one another. Some were slumped over, or asleep, others stared vacantly into space. As I continued down the hall, I noticed other residents who had on their TV sets for companionship, but appeared disinterested in the content of the shows. There were no visitors to be seen.

The home had an excellent nursing staff, well versed in the use of medications, and able to attend to a wide range of physical problems by literally racing from room to room. I asked the head nurse about the lack of visitors, and she replied, "It's really sad. A few of our patients are lucky, and have someone coming in once or twice a week, but many of them don't see any family or friends for weeks or months at a time. We have a fair number of people who are so old that they have out-lived every one of their family and friends, and their grandchildren have moved to other parts of the country. This is especially true of that group you saw coming in. They never go to occupational therapy like our more lively residents do, and they become steadily more demented as the years go on."

Dementia was indeed rampant in the building—both the slow kind just alluded to, and the more fulminating kind in Alzheimer's disease. Almost all of the patients I was asked to see, over a two-year period, were disoriented about the date and where they were, and many could not even give their own names. Typically, they were referred to me because they had struck out at staff members while being fed or bathed, and had developed a hostile attitude towards nurses.

I soon learned that it was useless to try to talk about these incidents, or anything else in the here and now. Their memory for recent events was nil, and I could find no present interest on which we could focus together. I knew, of course, that their memory for the distant past was much better, but it took a while to learn how to use this medical fact to advantage.

One day I was talking with a ninety-year-old woman of European extraction who had begun to have angry outbursts towards the nursing staff. She was unable to provide any explanation for this change of atti-tude, but along with it she had stopped going to occupational therapy, and confined herself to her room spending much of the time in bed. The staff feared a deepening of her mild dementia.

I asked if she had grown up in "the old country" and she began halt-ingly to describe how she had lived in a small cottage that was heated by a large fireplace in the living room. This led to some thoughts about her mother who tended the fireplace and also used it to bake bread for the family. She became more animated as she described her mother's baking techniques, and suddenly she climbed out of bed to show me, on the wall of her room, just how large the fireplace enclosure was. Bending over the imaginary hearth, she demonstrated how her mother rescued her finished product from the fire below so as not to get burned in the process. I thought to myself, "This woman is enjoying her psychiatric consultation more than any patient I've seen in years."

She sat in her chair then, and provided a fairly reasonable explanation for her pique with the nurses. The patient had married at age nineteen into a family belonging to a clan different from her own. She and her husband were very much in love but her mother-in-law never accepted her, refusing to call her by her first name, and always referring to her as "that woman." Her mother-in-law had also rallied other family members against her, making her husband's life miserable and often excluding both of them from family gatherings. The mother-in-law had three sisters all of who were deadly enemies of the patient, and one of them had recently moved into the same nursing home, and onto the same floor. The patient was enraged by the other woman's presence there, but couldn't tell the nurses about "such a private family matter." She had asked to be relocated to another floor, saying only that there was someone she didn't like on the floor. Her request had been refused because she wouldn't give any details. When they heard about the intense anger that was fueling her "dislike," the nurses quickly rearranged her room location and dining room hours to avoid any contact with her enemy. Good human contact with the nursing staff was restored, and she showed an immediate improvement in her mental state. She resumed reading the newspapers and her medication with Haldol was discontinued.

Using the same approach of finding an important special interest from the remote past for enjoyable conversation, I discovered that I would almost always see a reduction in dementia during consultations (except in the advanced Alzheimer patients). The people I saw were not hostile to me but, in fact, friendly. Their aggressive behaviors towards staff, however, continued for most of them with little or no abatement, so that they had to remain on Haldol.

It seemed clear to me that the aggressive patients were dealing with an unbearable rage brought about from their infirmities, and the massive loss of all their friends and family. Withdrawing had helped to rein in their hostility, and it only popped out from time to time, but it had the negative effect of depriving them of the care and concern that was available in the building. The overworked nursing staff simply did not have the time to provide them, on a daily basis, with the same kind of engagement as a visiting psychiatrist who had over a half-hour at his disposal. The pressure on staff to move on to the next patient was exposing the angry ones to repeated desertions throughout the day, which was the root cause of their aggressive outbursts.

Haldol could take the edge off their aggression, but it did nothing to prevent the daily build-up of more rage. Anti-depressant medication was of help for some but not for many. The only effective treatment was good human contact, which both mitigated the rage, and ameliorated dementia. Once again the superiority of the healing exchange of warmth over psychopharmacologic approaches was in evidence during the consultations. I learned early on to always pull up a chair to the bedside to indicate my intention to stay for a while. Introductions took place in the standing position to obtain better face-to-face and eye-to-eye contact, but the bedside chair spoke to an extended and unhurried visit. The missing visitor was their greatest need. For Alzheimer patients, the upright position sometimes had to be maintained throughout, especially in the terminal phase when the patient's regression had reached the two-month-old level, and close-up snout-to-snout contact was the only kind possible.

Why were there no visitors? After all, the nursing home in question took in members of every Faith, and over the years its residents had belonged to almost every parish and neighborhood in greater Washington. Surely the churches, at least, could have recruited a few of their members to visit with their own. But it didn't happen that way. Powerful unconscious forces were at work creating the same kind of internal resistance to involvement with these very elderly and lonely people as with the cancer victims.

They were living evidence that you could escape the fate of premature death, but at the cost of a massive wearing down of your body that shriveled up as if in anticipation of the final moment of death. The sight of the awesome destructive process they were undergoing was a powerful deterrent to visits from neighbors. As with the church groups, they were seemingly unaware that a friendly visit could be of help. And so, these abandoned humans were left to turn off their brains to cope with the impoverished state of rage in which they spent their final days.

If only some churches or charitable groups could have adopted small areas of this home on the hill to promote visits, but even more to foster a communal interest in upgrading the bleak surroundings. Some soft music and quiet conversation to silence the rancorous TV's for starters. The participants in such a program would have discovered a new dimension to their self-worth by helping their elderly counterparts to cope. The reduction in dementia alone would have provided unmistakable evidence for the value of their efforts.

The members of the wheelchair circle were so burned out and exhausted that they were rarely referred for assaults on the staff. They had somehow managed to hold on to life even though they appeared to be already in the grip of death. With the few whom I got to see it was wonderful to discover that they still had a spark of warmth that could be fanned into a glow by the presence of a visitor. Human life is indeed a very special state of being precisely because of our capacity to link up with one another, and feed each other emotionally.

Who is it that benefits the most from such a visit? The elderly resident clearly gets a lift that improves the function of a weary mind, but regular visits are needed to achieve more lasting change. A volunteer has the much more profound and durable experience of these encounters. She or he grows a bit so that the threat of death, or the id itself, becomes less ominous. Above all, there is a re-discovery of the basic secret of our human nature that we are here for the good of one another.

20

Healing our nine/eleven wounds

Before September the eleventh I had regarded the overcoming of prejudice as an ideal goal for human beings, perhaps even the pathway to a more refined civilization that lived under the Golden Rule. In the aftermath of September eleven, overcoming prejudice has become a necessary goal for our nation and the world. The front-page pictures of ferocious mobs in "neutral" Pakistan depicted a primitive horde with bared teeth. Their destructive drive pressures were of the raw cannibalistic kind. For us, the ruthless and wanton taking of human lives at the Pentagon and World Trade Center gave rise to a powerful surge of destructive energies that have been the source of stress disorders for many. When the destructive drives are on the rise sleep is disturbed and anxiety and depression invade the day. There is a sense of danger, along with a fear that our peaceful lives will never be the same again.

At present we are still engaged in the important task of strengthening the armed forces to convince enemies not to attack us. We see ourselves correctly as the victims of prejudice, but have to acknowledge the presence of a wide range of prejudices within our own borders. Doing something to change them may be the last good chance to avoid a global conflagration. Showing the rest of the world it can be done would demonstrate a moral and spiritual strength even more important than military power.

To heal an endangered world, we can lead the way by undertaking the healing of our own inner cities. The assassination of Dr. Martin

Luther King opened a gaping wound of prejudice between blacks and whites around the country, and also gave rise to the development of "attitudes" on both sides that have built a high wall of prejudice between the inner cities and suburbs. It's time for the wall to come down. If we can tear it down the rest of the world may begin to see us in a different light.

We have reached the point where the polarity between suburbanites and those within the city has ripened into a cold war. The very persons who could best help to heal the open violence in urban neighborhoods remain coldly aloof and afraid to venture there. A few churches have reached out across the great divide, but the loving energies of a vast multitude of suburban volunteers are needed to overcome rampant hatefulness. The fires of altruism are burning brightly within a new generation of high school and college students who can help their parents to overcome stranger anxiety. Together they could bring new warmth to the lives of parents and kids in the inner city, and help them to transform their surroundings. The "miracle of D.C.General" could be repeated in an American miracle of the inner cities, showing the rest of the world how to end violence between neighbors.

I grew up in World War Two with my freshman year in high school marred by a "sneak attack" on Pearl Harbor that also killed three thousand innocent people. By the end of the war I was a private in the Marine Corps infantry getting ready for the "landing" in Japan. I remember the wonderful patriotic fervor that united all of us to do something for our country, each in our own way. Every family was totally proud of its servicemen, and servicewomen. Many other women gained respect for doing "men's work" in defense plants, as "Rosie the Riviters." The war had a tragic ending in a human calamity, but like many others in the Army, Navy, Marine Corps, Coast Guard and Air Force, I was relieved that my own life had been spared. We're in just as much trouble now as then, maybe more so. This time we might be the victims of a nuclear attack, and city streets may become a war zone for suicidal bombings.

It hasn't been as easy to develop the same kind of national support for the wars in Iraq and against terrorists as we did in World War Two. These have been different kinds of war, more "high tech", and requiring less fighters. This time, however, most of us on the home front still have a chance to play a much greater part. The attack we have experienced so far has been an attack on our national culture and our national spirit. We can actualize the great American Dream, and Dr. Martin Luther King's dream, by helping the poor to climb out of the depths of poverty and squalor to create newer and better lives for themselves.

In World War Two, a great national organization emerged, the USO, to give civilians a chance to share their warmth and hospitality with servicemen and women at canteens around the world. We now need a new kind of service organization, a mighty crusade of volunteers from the suburbs to descend on the inner cities, and share their warmth with the people there. This has already begun with the various suburban church groups that have adopted inner city churches to create a channel for donations of furniture, books, clothing, and also for getting to know one another better. Volunteer initiatives could be especially effective in hospitals that treat the poor and the sick, in schools and in public housing projects. In many parts of the country doctor volunteers are running free medical clinics for the needy. These might also serve as valuable centers for joint action between suburbanites and inner city residents.

Our hope on September the Eleventh that we might find some survivors in the ruins of the World Trade Center and Pentagon ended in bitter disappointment. There were none, but there are lots of survivors in wretched condition in the inner cities. Lending them a hand in a person-to-person way would heal our reputation of selfishness in some parts of the Arab world. By overcoming our prejudice and reaching out to destitute neighbors we would also gain the increase in loving energies necessary to heal residual stress disorders. The healing of the inner cities would not be a one-way street. Doing for others in dire straits would bring on their healing gratitude, providing a tonic for our health and self-esteem.

21

The existence and functions of the soul

Early in this story about a doctor's experience with healing we found ourselves in a very unlikely place, a public hospital for the mentally ill where there was very little healing going on. To conclude it we must revisit that hospital where the miracle of D.C.General took place in order to have a further look at its most important lesson. Practically speaking, the most obvious conclusion to be drawn from the events at D.C.General is that schizophrenics are hurt by isolation from other people and helped by the immediate restoration of good human contact. Of greater importance is the fact that the healing at D.C.General provided new medical evidence for the existence and functions of a spiritual component to our human nature, namely the human soul.

Twentieth Century psychiatry was dominated by Freud's three dimensional model of the mind: an ego or organized executive portion, a superego comprised of a conscience and set of ideals, and an id, or seething cauldron of relentless sexual and aggressive drive energies. Freud derived this model from his work with people suffering from the neuroses—non-psychotic illnesses like hysteria, obsessions, compulsions, sexual perversions and personality disorders. In his 1924 paper, "The Ego and the Id," he clarified the relationship between the ego and the id. He credited the ego with playing an active role in warding off the id through a set of defense mechanisms, but in all of these, the id itself remained unchanged.

Freud was fascinated by the illness of schizophrenia and used the richly detailed autobiography of a schizophrenic patient to try to shed some new light on the disease. His paper, "The Case of Schreber", showed Freud's genius and humanity in attempting to make some sense out of Judge Schreber's catastrophic mental downfall. His conviction that we would one day solve the mystery of schizophrenia helped me to keep on task in times of doubt and despair about reaching this goal.

In our experience at D.C. General it was clear that schizophrenia was the illness par excellence for the study of the id. For most of our patients a boiling over of the id had indeed obliterated the ego. Our patients had been telling us for years that they were no longer real persons, and had become robots or mechanical people. Many of them believed that everyone in the world had undergone the same transformation. We learned that this strange perception of self and others was due to a deep withdrawal from the world that had cut off their ability to share caring feelings with other people. And from this we deduced that there was a portion of our loving energies that actually bound us together as a species with one another, and that this connectedness must remain unbroken for rationality to exist. We had stumbled on a really remarkable part of our human nature, a bonding power of our inner warmth that could act as an antidote for the destructive drives, rein them in and make them manageable once more. The presence in each of us of a resource that could directly modify the id in others and in ourselves called for the recognition of a higher power in our model of the mind, a fourth dimension, more powerful than the other three, with a range of special and unique functions of its own. This fourth dimension is clearly the spiritual entity known as the soul.

The possession of a soul has been a central dogma of almost all religions. It is usually seen as a spiritual component that is infused into the embryo by an All-Loving God, monitors the relationship between God and humans, and survives after death for a reunion with God. The existence of the soul has been the focus for heated debate between believers in God, and non-believers. If the soul is looked at strictly from a perspective of the medical evidence at D.C.General it emerges as a very refined portion of our loving instincts that can subjugate the destructive instincts. The soul is a healing resource of great value with an enormous potential for the future development of a more peaceful human race. In this light the soul is a unifying concept with room for both believers in God and non-believers. The linkage of one human being with another through their capacity to share care and concern is the function of the soul that supports both rationality and healing. In retrospect, getting through to schizophrenics at D.C.General was facilitated by a network of connections between staff and patients that had simply been idle and only needed a little boost of loving energies to be re-started. None of us had anticipated that there would be a hunger for relatedness to other humans in every one of our patients that would allow them to heal the overload of powerful destructive urges that had caused their deep withdrawal. They shared their inner warmth with one another all day long so that the tiny nursing staff that had concerned our consultant, Dr. Jack Ewalt, could easily manage the challenges of a totally unlocked hospital. The soul is an inner spirit or animus that gives purposefulness to our being. The presence of the soul is sometimes felt as a deep yearning to share our warmth with others, or as a calling to greater achievement. We are born with a noble purpose, to seek to perfect ourselves by modifying our destructive urges and infantile selves in order to become more loving to other human beings, and in appropriate ways to ourselves.

The soul provides the bedrock that is the basis for good self-esteem. We are able to do something that other animals cannot do, to modify our destructive drives by an act of the will to share our warmth. We have a higher degree of control over our base instincts, particularly the destructive drives. Of this we can be justly proud. The more that we can use our loving energies to help others the better our self-esteem. As a spiritual entity the soul can make its healing and inspiring presence available to many people at the same time as we have seen in the case of religious leaders like Ghandi and Pope John Paul Two, or scientists like Einstein and Freud.

A good example of the survival power of the soul was the experience I have already described at the funeral of my colleague and friend Dr. John Kuhn. I felt very sad as we followed his casket out of the church, thinking we had lost such a good man. Suddenly it was as though he were walking beside me, and saying "Why don't you go over to that home for AIDS patients and take my place there." I've been going there ever since. His spirit clearly lives on in the minds of all that knew him.

Freud was one of the first to recognize that human beings take their parents inside after their death and remodel their personalities along the lines of a deceased mother or father. This event can occur so quickly that it may be better explained by the survival of the soul of the deceased than by the also true psychoanalytic concept of identification with the lost object. I know that I immediately began to advise my father on the selection of his clothes and help him to plan his day after the death of my mother. It was not long afterward that colleagues began to comment on my ability to function in a maternal way with patients. And not too much later that I felt that urging inside, coming from my mother, to learn to speak rationally with acutely disturbed schizophrenics.

There are many single people who are saddened by their failure to produce offspring. If they have lived a life of helping others they can take consolation in that their loving energies became a part of these persons and will be passed on to future generations. The souls of nuns, priests and single lay people live on in the minds and hearts of those to whom they have been close.

Sometimes the healing operation of the soul hits a snag, as with a rebellious teenage son or daughter, a hard-nosed boss or an unruly subordinate. To get through to them and change their disposition one has to first be able to feel what is going on inside them. To accomplish this another function of the soul is necessary, namely empathy.

Empathy is the deepest form of good human contact and goes well beyond the simple sharing of inner warmth between two people. When we are able to perceive what causes pain inside another, we bring it into ourselves where it is exposed to the healing love drive. As we communicate these events by word or deed to someone in pain, they experience a resonance that doubles the soothing effect of our empathy. Two souls become united through a sharing of inner warmth, and pain becomes more tolerable. Without the empathic response, healing love is only passively present in those two souls, like information in our memory banks. It only becomes meaningful when we put it to use.

The concept of empathy includes our ability to be aware of any and every kind of feeling in another. In some platonic relationships, there is an almost one hundred percent concordance between the inner life of two people, much like that of identical twins. These individuals have no secrets from each other, can readily engage in the most intimate conversations, and find their special friendship to be a source of strength. They are soul mates without sexual interaction who may not even meet so frequently, but when they do, they come away renewed, and refreshed in spirit by the exchange of healing love.

A touching example of the growth potential in such a relationship was portrayed in the movie "The Postman". A painfully shy young man meets the world-renowned poet, Pablo Neruda, on an important day for both of them. It is the youth's first day in his new job as a mail carrier, and the day the poet arrives in exile at a small island fishing village. The young man hardly dares to speak out of awe for his distinguished customer. He is fascinated by the latter's ability to win the ardor of women from all over the world, and scrutinizes Neruda's loving relationship with his wife with intense interest. A friendship soon develops in which they share their appreciation of nature's beauty around the island. The poet discovers the rudiments of a poetic gift in his friend and carefully cultivates it. He also teaches his pupil how to overcome his shyness with women so that he is able to woo and wed the girl of his dreams. Following his benefactor's footsteps, the young man becomes an ardent Communist, and is killed in a riot as he is about to be honored by the Party for his poetic contributions to their cause.

As we watch the movie, we become aware of an unusual advance in personal development that has taken place in the hero's life. No longer a trembling swain of few words, he successfully enters an intense and intimate love relationship that produces a son, and clearly has the power to survive his death. He becomes able to translate his sensitive perception of nature's beauty into words, and to use his speech aggressively in support of his political beliefs. To achieve such a spurt in his growth, which takes him way beyond anything we might have expected from the early moments of the film, a powerful loving influence must have been at work. It was the result of two souls blending in a platonic relationship that generated an enormous amount of healing love. The young man's involvement in a heterosexual love relationship later augmented this.

The end of the movie reveals the enduring quality of both of these relationships. The widow goes about her work contentedly, bolstered by her persistent love for her late husband and her maternal love for their son. Before his death, the young man had heard nothing from his friend until he received an impersonal letter from the poet-politico's secretary requesting some of the belongings he had left behind. The letter caused a painful narcissistic hurt but failed to alter his conviction that his friend would one-day return and resume their warm relationship. As the ending shows, he was correct in his expectation that their mutual fondness would last. The poet and his wife do return for a reunion with their friend and are shocked and saddened to learn of his death. When the inner warmth of two souls becomes actively engaged in a platonic relationship, it acquires an extraordinary power to survive.

Intuition is a fairly close relative to empathy in the family of soul functions. It is the fast track of the mind that enables one to know something without resorting to conscious reasoning. We use it often to size up others in a first meeting so that we may deal with them in the most effective way. Intuition is probably the product of information about the world, and people in it, that has been passed on to us through countless generations of ancestors. It would thus be the result of knowledge that has been circulated through migrations of the soul after death. Intuition becomes a guideline for conduct in a wide range of situations. Saying the right thing in the right way and time can reach deeply into the soul of another and galvanize it into action during a crisis. The healing of people who were undergoing the torture of treatment-resistant depressions, in Chap. 13, gave an especially good example of this soul function in action. In each case the doctor's spontaneous, uncharacteristic and intuitive act was the perfect medicine for restoring hope. It showed the linkage function of the soul operating with surgical precision. A doctor's intuitive response to a patient's intuitive message changed the very self of both, producing a healing interaction.

How often do we hear it said that something done on a hunch produced a financial gain or personal triumph? Psychological studies at Duke University detailed in Doctor J.B.Rhyne's book, "The Reach of Mind", documented the existence of a capacity for extrasensory perception that was rudimentary for some but quite well developed in a number of people. It may be that intuition is still a work in progress for the human race, a part of the soul that is becoming more refined through further human experience in the healing of one another.

Intuition is also an example of another important achievement of the soul, the power of human beings to go way beyond the expected normal limits for human performance. Doctors are very familiar with this phenomenon. They see it every day in the accomplishments of patients who are able to survive well beyond the established prognosis for their stage of cancer, or every other kind of life-threatening illness. The incurable alcoholic whose disease has left him groveling in the gutter may suddenly escape from the shadow of death and develop a whole new life for himself in AA.

The constant shattering of world records in every sport attests to a burning desire in human beings that emanates from the soul and pushes athletes onward in their quest to go beyond. It was once thought by many doctors that the great Glenn Cunningham's record for a mile run in four minutes and four seconds represented a biological limit that could not be surpassed. The goal of a four-minute mile was considered out of the question until Roger Bannister accomplished the feat in 1952. Since then there have been many runners who keep lowering the barrier even further. When I think of the unique accomplishment of the D.C.General nursing staff in unlocking a public mental hospital for the acutely disturbed and discarding the use of restraints I often refer to them as the four-minute milers of psychiatry. Their extraordinary feat remains unsurpassed by other mental hospitals to this day.

The Soul is the agency of the mind that urges us onward in all things to do our best, and be the best. When it accomplishes this task in any given group of people they develop a wonderful attitude about their membership in the group. We call it esprit de corps, a can-do spirit that propels a whole body of people towards greater achievement and a closer friendship with one another. I have had the good fortune of being in six such organizations at critical junctures in my life. In temporal sequence they were: my High School, Regis in New York; the U.S.Marine Corps in World War Two; an Internship in internal medicine at Georgetown; Fellowship in psychiatry at the Beth Israel Hospital in Boston during the Camelot years; the psychiatric staff of D.C.General in the miracle years; and The Order of Malta in their annual pilgrimages to Lourdes.

The Soul has a very sensitive relationship to the existence of beauty, maintaining a constant lookout for the beautiful whether in persons, places or things. Gazing at the sudden sight of a snow-capped mountain range, as members of The Order of Malta do on arrival at Lourdes, the soul takes it deeply inside and nourishes itself. It gets filled with the emotions of awe and joy. Listening to a well-played symphony the soul experiences an inner peace. William Congreve said it best in 1697: "Music has charms to sooth the savage breast." When the soul feeds on beautiful sights and sounds it has a quieting effect on the destructive drives. The collection of loving energies that comprise the soul is truly the most beautiful part of the mind and it resonates harmoniously with beauty in the outside world whenever and wherever it is perceived.

The important place of beauty in our lives is the well-spring of creativity. An artist reaches deeply within to share emotional stirrings about a scene that permits the re-creation of a portion of nature. If his or her painting succeeds in capturing nature's splendor it will arrest our attention and elicit a joyful response. The soul experiences a double pleasure both from the beauty of the artist's work and the fact that it was produced by one of us. Artistic masterpieces are a valuable source of pride in our human nature. For those of us who are short on painting talent other creative urges can also permit the cultivation of things that are beautiful or useful from within ourselves, enhancing our self-esteem. The wide range of arts and crafts, writing, gardening, interior decoration and personal grooming all offer creative outlets. We take pride in these endeavors and they keep the soul well fortified with loving energies. Even in our sleep it guards against the intrusion of the destructive drives through dreams. The soul is able to harness the energy of the destructive drives and put it to work for loving purposes in the procedure called sublimation by Freud. Infantile urges to smear feces on the person or property of people who are despised get transformed in the soul into use of the hands to produce artistic works of beauty.

Human beings are free to choose their own behaviors as far as loving and hating are concerned. In this respect the sharing of inner warmth differs from other systems of medical healing such as the clotting mechanism or the immune response, for these are automatic in their operation. The sharing of inner warmth requires an act of volition—a willingness to share our love even with people who are suffering from an overload of the destructive drives. Freedom of the will sometimes permits terrible atrocities to be committed that are cited as a flaw in our human nature. But the fact that inner warmth needs a human decision to be set in motion has a profoundly beneficial effect on the soul. It strengthens willpower as we experience the good that a voluntary act can accomplish.

Willpower is the motor of the soul, a sheer determination to over-come the destructive drives within others, and in ourselves. It is the driving force behind outreach to the poor, the sick, and society's out-casts. Willpower operates in the steely resolve to survive and prevail in the face of adverse life circumstances. It is precisely because we have made a decision to share our warmth that the soul grows and willpower becomes stronger.

Marriage is a precious institution, at once human and divine, that draws heavily on the soul for a successful outcome. The guidelines for the sharing of loving energies laid out in the wedding ceremony under-score the role of the soul as the principal actor in the marital project. The essential spirituality of marriage is further attested to by the requirement of almost every religion that God be a third party partici-pant in the marriage contract. An All-Loving God is seen as having a vital interest in procreation and preservation of the integrity of families, and God also imposes exclusivity on the sexual relationship to further these purposes. When the childbearing period is over the sexual rela-tionship becomes even more important as a source of spiritual and bodily health, and pleasure.

Sexual intercourse provides an opportunity for a unique and pro-found sharing of inner warmth that is at once both sensual and spiri-tual. The spirituality comes from the endowment of the act with God's purposes, and the fact that basic differences between a man and woman (anatomic, biological, hormonal and emotional) have to be overcome for lovemaking to be successful. All four of these gender factors operate to create separate ways of approaching sex for the couple. In summary, men tend to proceed more quickly, and women more slowly. Married couples have to work together to understand and adapt to these differ-ences. By doing so they enhance their spirituality. Gender prejudice is overcome and the love drives become less self-centered, and more tuned in to the otherness of the beloved. The intense exchange of caring energies joins two bodies into one that overflows with loving feelings. There is also a union of two souls, making soul mates of a man and woman. After the childbearing period intercourse still has the profoundly spiritual purpose of strengthening the exchange of loving energies between men and women.

A lot of marriages in Washington and everyplace these days are shared by couples with busy and quite separate careers. My wife's weekends and many nights are devoted to serving her clients at the Washington Fine Properties, LLC. Her goal is always to find the perfect house for them and they become her good friends both during and after the process. Every few weeks we realize that we have begun to have a shortfall of time for intimate conversation. There is a remedy for this problem called the getaway, a twenty-four hour instant cure for marital inertia. Heading for the Ashby Inn in nearby Paris, Va. we stop at the Red Fox Inn in Middleburg, Va. for lunch and some shopping. Then it's fifteen more minutes to the Ashby Inn where proprietors John and Roma Sherman await us for some talk about politics, both local and national. In the Fall and Winter two armchairs by a crackling fire in the bedroom fireplace rekindle the warm energies of the soul. A walk down a country road along the foothills of the Blue Ridge Mountains completes the escape from Washington. Spring and Summer call for visits to the perennial garden, breakfasts and suppers on the outdoor patio, and relaxation on the bedroom balcony overlooking the first range of the Blue Ridge. The return home is accompanied by the kind of lasting enjoyment that only the soul can produce.

Marriages thrive on two other important operations of the soul, the generation of laughter and further development of a sense of humor. Laughter is the safety valve of the soul, a reliable outlet for inner tension, and frequent healing event for marital strife. (Remember how it quieted the lid-man's murderous impulses.) Most married couples quickly learn to laugh together about a lot of things: the lousy weather, the otherwise annoying shortcomings of some of their friends, and pretty soon about their own flaws. When they become able to laugh at themselves they achieve a triumph over narcissism that is rewarding. By openly acknowledging their mistakes they become more honest in their self-appraisal, and avoid the accumulation of guilt.

The soul is the most precious asset of our human nature and deserves the very best of care. As in every human activity the strength of the soul can be increased through exercise. We guard our physical health through a determination to watch our diet and engage in daily exercise. The same kind of commitment can be made to the soul through the frequent practice of spiritual exercise. Finding forms of spiritual exercise that will work for both believers in God and non-believers will be our next topic.

22

Spiritual exercise to strengthen the soul

Spiritual exercise has been a wonderful human institution for a long time. Its purpose is to seek a refinement of our loving energies so that they become less self-serving and increase in their power to heal the destructive drives in others and in us. The concept of spiritual exercise encompasses a wide range of methods that have emerged from a number of different sources. We have already considered some of the more active forms of spiritual exercise such as marriage, intimate relationships and volunteer work with society's outcasts. What follows is a look at other forms that are more cerebral.

Four hundred years ago, St. Ignatius Loyola, that great Christian warrior and founder of the Society of Jesus, designed a 30-day spiritual workout to toughen the religious spines of his followers. His regimen was based on the idea that human beings could try, in a systematized way, to become more like their Creator. There have been many subsequent programs with the same goal, including Alcoholics Anonymous and the other coalitions of self and God, to fight addictions. These self-help organizations have widened their spiritual embrace with the concept of a Higher Power as the motivating force for non-believers in God. The Higher Power is a spiritual entity with loving and healing energies that overcome self-destructive behavior and provide emotional growth. It is the same as the concept of the soul derived from the healing of schizophrenics at D.C.General. While the program of St. Ignatius is suitable training for sainthood or running in a spiritual marathon, there are other kinds of spiritual exercise, like AA, that can strengthen the souls of both believers in God and non-believers.

Psychoanalysis is actually a form of spiritual exercise and as a treatment its patients include many that are atheists, or agnostics, as well as members of the religious right. Its goals of removing the neurotic elements in a person's life and increasing self-understanding enhance and help to refine the loving energies of the soul. The shared warmth between analyst and patients is really one of its greatest therapeutic assets. Psychoanalysts will usually acknowledge how important their personal warmth is to success in the project, but they hesitate to speak openly of this. The ability to get through and provide an exchange of warmth is indeed rarely addressed in the training institutes, for fear of appearing unscientific. Increasingly, in modern years, psychoanalysis has focused on all the residuals of infantile behavior still present. This shift was noted by a number of world famous analysts who participated in the Jenny Waelder Hall Symposium in Baltimore in 1964. Several of them suggested that when the analysis of a person's childhood neurosis has been completed, they would recommend beginning the analysis of their narcissism, with its self-centered infantile components. At the conclusion of a successful psychoanalysis it is customary to encourage the person being analyzed to practice self-analysis at regular intervals. This means to allow one's thoughts to flow with complete freedom, while an observing part of the mind monitors them to see where they may lead in the search for a greater self-understanding. There will be no analyst sitting behind to help out, but he or she may sometimes show up in the flow also, often to assist, other times to be targeted for anger or infantile wishes. There is only one analyst present now, with full responsibility for the improvement of himself or herself.

For those who have been analyzed, a regular period of meditation on the intrusions of the infantile into their daily lives would strengthen the soul. Free association means allowing one's thoughts to flow without any censoring. It can be a very humbling experience because it requires us to look at things we don't like about ourselves, such as impatience, anger, envy or prejudice. When we can allow ourselves to come face to face with the infantile and still harmful underside of our nature, we expose it to a loving side that stimulates personal growth. Doing an honest review of our infantile moments of the day in a quiet, thoughtful way is a key element of most kinds of spiritual exercise.

Alcoholics Anonymous is a very successful form of group spiritual exercise that also requires its members to focus on their infantile foibles. It draws heavily on the linkage function of the soul and the sharing of personal warmth for its effectiveness. At the outset, new members make a commitment to attend daily meetings for at least ninety days, and several meetings a week thereafter. Spiritual exercise means making a commitment to your soul to allow some time for a contemplative engagement with it on as many days each week as possible. Believers in God and non-believers can both acknowledge that there is a special part of our nature that calls for us to be more caring towards one another and needs our frequent attention.

For many years after my own analysis I practiced the recommended form of self-analysis and was satisfied with the results. I thought of myself as a firm believer in God, with a faith inherited from my parents and from countless generations of Protestant and Catholic forbears who preceded them. My mother's parents were staunch Lutherans and my father's just as devoted to Catholicism. I did my reaching out to God in Church and it never occurred to me to include The Almighty in my efforts at self-improvement through meditation.

During the remarkable days at D.C.General I began to think there is something uncanny going on here, something in defiance of our knowledge about schizophrenia. I didn't dare to think of it as due to the intervention of God but I was attracted to the AA notion of a Higher Power at work. Changes in schizophrenic patients were coming about so rapidly that I could find no human explanation. I began to think that our patients and staff had been possessed by a Higher Power with an extraordinary healing potential. Working with the medically ill at Beth Israel Hospital in Boston had already made me aware that the simple sharing of inner warmth between a doctor and uncooperative patient could lead to a major improvement in health. At D.C.General it became apparent that this healing warmth was present in every human being, even coldly aloof schizophrenics who had been living in a world of their own. Now, many years later, as I have begun to reflect on the lessons of D.C.General, I have been more and more struck by the need for a better explanation of the events that took place there. Most of our patients fell into one of three categories on admission: they were either openly violent, seething with rage and potentially violent, or so totally withdrawn from the world that they couldn't do violence. Almost all were withdrawn from one another, and from the staff. And yet every one of us, patients and staff alike, had an inner warmth that allowed us to join up with one another, and had the almost immediate effect of calming violent urges. What was this healing inner warmth? Where did it come from? We could start by saying that maybe it came about through a process of the gradual evolution of a nucleus of loving energies that got started in primitive men and women and slowly acquired a healing function. Indeed maybe it did start that way. But that still doesn't tell us why there would be a part of our loving energies that joins us together with one another as a species, gives rise to rationality, and has an extraordinary power to modify the destructive drives.

It seems to me that what we had learned from the healing of schizophrenics at D.C.General cast a significant new light on our origin as a species. We were creatures with an unusually powerful brain that seemed to have an unlimited capacity for new discoveries. And yet this wonderful tool for advancement could not function properly unless we were in a caring mode towards one another. Our loving energies, meanwhile, also had very special powers and a limitless potential for growth. They could directly modify the destructive drives in others, and in us, bringing an inner peace to both. The result of these triumphs over hatred was an increase and further refinement of the loving energies. A likely purpose to our being emerges from these events, namely that we are here for the good of one another. I find this to be medical evidence strongly supportive of my own faith that we had our origin as a species in an All-Loving God. I also believe that our extraordinary, healing inner warmth comes from the actual presence of God within the souls of each of us. This is the bottom line for the conviction of so many that human life is sacred. It is also the reason why people can go way beyond their expected limitations in times of severe distress, or in their zeal for the discovery of new knowledge. The Higher Power is our love for our fellow man, which is the essence of the human soul and issues forth from our common origin in an All-Loving God. It has an amazing power to heal the destructive drives as seen in the case of AA, or in the miracle of D.C.General where it produced an almost instant modification of the id.

As a believer in God, I consider the soul to be that part of ourselves where both God and we humans reside and interact. For this reason my own spiritual exercise through meditation takes the form of a dialogue with God. Those who do not believe in God can carry out the same kind of review of their infantile moments with their Higher Power, an ideal part of the soul that urges us to make our loving energies more readily available to all of our fellow humans. We have good reason to pay homage to the soul through the frequent practice of spiritual exercise. It may be the answer to survival for the human race.

The soul has been glorified in so many hymns and spirituals. "This little light of mine, Lord let it shine, All across the world I'm going to let it shine, Let it shine." Many have tried to give the soul a specific bodily placement, usually in the heart, as in "I've got the love of Jesus down in my heart, down in my heart." A deep bodily placement is appropriate because the soul, as a spiritual entity, resides in every part of the human body. People in crisis may not only display extraordinary courage but they can also muster unusual degrees of bodily strength to cope with external danger, if their souls are robust. One of the most intense forms of human anxiety is called fragmentation anxiety because it involves a fear that the body may fly apart into pieces, or simply collapse and fall apart. People sometimes refer to it as a fear that they are going to explode. A healthy soul provides the greatest protection against this type of anxiety because it increases a person's conviction about the cohesiveness of their bodily self.

If one accepts the notion that God is somewhere present in each of us, or that there is a special and finer kind of love in the soul, then it should be possible to establish a dialogue between the more human aspect of ourselves and this divine or special portion of the soul. The dialogue requires only some quiet time for self-reflection and is a wonderful way to start and end each day. It can be resumed at any opportune moment, in an easy chair before the TV set (turned off), or behind an office door closed to afford a brief shelter from the outside world. It may proceed aboard a bus or Metro train, where observations of the needs or contentment of fellow passengers can help fuel the process.

How can we have a dialogue with God, or with a Higher Power when we don't have the slightest idea of what Either may look like? It helps to be able to conjure up the picture of another human being, and some are able to do this by thinking of Jesus Christ and drawing on His image from their childhood prayer books. Christ was indeed fully human as well as Divine and he must have experienced all of the human temptations and emotional shortcomings. We ought to be able to feel completely comfortable in His loving presence and be able to engage in a person-to-person dialogue. If it is hard to picture Jesus, or a Higher Power, for this purpose there is another way of experiencing them in a human form. Since Both exist in every person we have only to think of a good friend with whom we have felt completely at ease and begin our review of the day with that individual. The one selected may be a man or woman. If God or the Higher Power have a gender it must be both. Someone of the opposite sex who has been a platonic friend would be an excellent spiritual companion. Such a person could bring a special warmth that has already been enjoyed, and be able to listen carefully and with care to our trials and tribulations. Of course the choice might also be a kindred spirit of the same sex. So we can begin our meditation with some thoughts about an old friend for whom we have the greatest respect and love, knowing that our friend is acting as a stand-in for God or a Higher Power. This is the warm-up phase of spiritual exercise. A good opener might be to imagine ourselves on a walk with this friend enjoying some of the wonderful sights of nature. The memory of inspirational vistas could help us to do this. The awesome beauty of a rugged mountain range, the restful beauty of verdant pastures, or the quintessential beauty of a rose in bloom would serve as a tonic for the soul. Poets have addressed this phenomenon in so many artful ways of their own. I sometimes begin my warm-up by recalling a few lines written by Sidney Lanier in his "Ode to the Marshes of Glynn" at Sea Island in Georgia. He describes the beauty of the marshes as he came to know them while recuperating from an illness acquired as a prisoner of the North in the Civil War. A man of great cultural attainment, Lanier fought on the side of the South and was able to walk home from Gettysburg to Georgia even while suffering from tuberculosis. His soul achieved a remarkable triumph over a disabling medical illness. It was indeed a winning of good out of infinite pain. The lives of great men inspire both believers and non-believers.

In a campaign speech in West Virginia, President Kennedy alluded to Robert Frost's description of a man who feasted on nature's beauty to fortify himself for a journey, and the task of meeting his responsibilities in life. Frost describes a lone traveler pondering a snowfall at the outset of a challenging day. We are not alone on our trek to nightfall, but share the way with the very Creator of our remarkable world, or with a loving soul.

A true sense of companionship with God, or a Higher Power, can only develop when we are able to hold the most honest and intimate form of conversation with them. Like every other human achievement, it takes practice and exercise to get there. We are talking about a kind of exchange that is completely open, devoid of secrets, and absolutely free. Whatever comes to mind on a subject must be put on the table for ourselves and companion to share. Even the most intimate of human conversations, as between husband and wife, penitent and confessor, or analysand and psychoanalyst are never so free. In this type of discourse, every false pretension, all the hidden motives and rationalizations for our behavior, must be allowed to rise to the surface for inspection and correction. The grown-up self has its final moment of triumph over the infantile.

Believers in God may begin with the acknowledgement of God's greatness and goodness to emphasize the incomparable disparity between His/Her limitless perfection and our own imperfect condition. We are mortal, and even the occasional genius among us can accomplish only so much through mental effort. The work of creation itself bespeaks a fantastic mind that endures through all the ages. In the presence of such a Spiritual Power, a state of humility is appropriate and necessary to the whole tone of our conversation with God. We have much to be humble about, including many of the thoughts, feelings, and experiences of the preceding day or night. People who do not believe in God could probably say pretty much the same thing vis-a-vis their Higher Power.

It isn't necessary to engage in mental self-flagellation. If we simply expose our human frailties and proclivity for self-deception to an all-loving part of ourselves we can study these shortcomings together. As already suggested, spiritual exercise has much in common with the technique that Freud discovered for the cure of hysteria and subsequently molded into a method of treatment for all personality flaws: psychoanalysis. Spiritual exercises, however, go beyond psychoanalysis in their therapeutic aim, for they seek to heal the split in the mind between its adult and infantile portions, and to restore the human soul to a full accord with its Creator, or with our highest ideals.

What a difference it can make in our lives when we finally come to accept as fact the reality of a Timeless and Very Special Portion of our nature that must be given first priority throughout the day. The ubiquitous problem of impatience can then be subjected to thorough overhaul. Think of how much anger we generate over those who impede our use of the precious commodity of time. The slow-poke clerk who delays our departure from a store may be either scorned as stupid or dismissed as a willful obstructionist who delights in mis-serving his customers. The same for the slow driver whose lightness of foot deprives us of five seconds. How important we must be to deserve such deference to our needs, and to attach such an enormous value to our time.

"What's your hurry?" asks our thoughtful Inner-companion. The gentle query invites self-reflection. The hurry-worry is a wonderful marker for spiritual intervention. Our time is a gift from God, or a de facto possession of all of us. We do not own it, but simply share in its allotment with every other living being. We are joined with them by a common purpose, which is to live for the good of one another. The person behind the counter or the inept motorist provides a fresh opportunity to enjoy our mission in the world. We are not kings or queens, but only faithful servants. Knowing and accepting this, we are immune to insult and needless, debilitating anger.

The question, "What's your hurry?" is an example of the kind of dialogue that can occur as we review our thoughts and feelings of the day in spiritual exercise. The calm, dispassionate, and loving tone of this dialogue is a welcome contrast to the gruff or demeaning exchange sometimes associated with the voice of conscience. As we respond to such helpful questions, an overly strict, stern, or even cruel conscience can be modified, and pointless guilt will be reduced. Once in a while, the spiritual exchange may include a prodding "There you go again," which is more likely to provoke a chuckle than a Reaganesque put-down. We have to learn to laugh at ourselves to overcome the crippling illness of exaggerated self-importance.

President Carter provided another splendid marker for spiritual reflection when he drew public attention to the phenomenon of lust in the heart. Lust is a mental event with an unmistakable physical component. Secret sexual longings towards someone other than one's spouse are worthy of note when accompanied by a roving eye, or regularly indulged in as a fallback source of sexual pleasure. The harmless kinds generally do not remain a secret very long, but those that are persistent and occult deserve to be shared with the Wonderful Partner of our secret life. They are usually out of sync with mature sexuality and may be a sign of marital discord. It is better to be completely honest with ourselves about lust than to act it out in destructive fashion. The spiritual arena is the one forum where total candor is always possible. Jealousy, envy, anger, and sexual urges are simply parts of the human condition, which deserve an admixture with God's love or the highest aspirations of the soul.

The contribution to the dialogue that comes from these sources can take other forms besides inspirational questions. A sudden vignette from childhood may emerge casting a new light on a problem of adulthood, allowing us to view the offensive behavior of another with a whole new perspective. How petty our mortal concerns can be when they are carefully studied. Insight itself comes from God or from the highest and finest portion of the mind. Through insight we progress to gratitude, a state of perfect harmony within the soul.

Gratitude flows from a full appreciation of gifts that have been received. It is a contentment that is all encompassing. Freud's British colleague, Dr. Melanie Klein, described this emotion as one of the earliest feeling states of an infant as it experiences the fullness of a mother's love at her breast or simply in her arms. Gratitude is an antidote for infantile rage, and thus a core element of our humanity. When gratitude is present, envy is discarded. The pressure to get more and have more, sooner and in a hurry, is relieved so that anger is no longer necessary. Gratitude is indeed a precious state of the emotions.

Spiritual exercise can be carried on throughout the day in many other ways besides the study of our infantile flaws. As we stand above a beautiful valley and look out over the rolling hills that form its walls, a moment of perfect spirituality is possible. We have come upon a magnificent part of the world and are enthralled by its beauty. Our gratitude for this moment of experience is complete and we realize that this is what gratitude is all about, a thankfulness for our very existence in a world that has inspired our souls. Such a brief interval of time can tell us all we need to know, who we are and why we are here, and why we can rejoice, simply to be a living part of the world's Greatness. When we allow our hearts to swell with this feeling, we are Columbus, the discoverers of a New World more bountiful by far than the one in which we live our daily lives. We can reenter the old with new confidence and hope.

It is thus that the conquest of time is achieved. The most painful part of a doctor's work involves the care of those whose life faces premature termination. But does it really matter if we live one more day or ten or ten years? Compared with eternity, the normal life span becomes a second, indeed a millisecond. What really counts is that we have given of the goodness in our hearts. This is our gift to the gene pool of mankind. It requires no offspring to be complete. We can take comfort in the knowledge that we have shared our warmth with others. They are better for it and we are ready to do so again until the end. With this in mind, a doctor can give his all, his own inner strength and love, expressed in his touch, words, and eye contact for the doctor and patient are also one. The same may be said for all of us. We have shared in the very special nature of human existence, and we await the common fate of death. The soul survives to go on helping family and friends, and hoping for a happy reunion with our Creator. We don't know what form this reunion may take, but we can accept our ignorance in gratitude for all that we have been able to know. The soul guarantees our immortality by guiding the investment of our loving energies into others who in turn are able to impart this best portion of ourselves to future generations.

Carrying out the mandates of the soul is the most basic kind of spiritual exercise. The soul drives us to do more and be more, in essence to function at our best. When we are at our best, the soul rewards us with the emotion of joy in a reminder that by living up to our potential, we fulfill the promise of our creation and move ever closer to oneness with God, or towards an ideal state of human existence. The uniquely pleasurable feeling of joy is associated in most Christians' minds with the two great religious seasons of Christmas and Easter. In fact, it can be a daily occurrence for people of every belief or non-belief if the soul is getting enough spiritual exercise. Driving across town to help out in a halfway house or homeless shelter, a dreary trip becomes the Skyline Drive. A friendly nod to a passing stranger may provide a moment of joy for two. Holding hands in an AA meeting and thinking how far one has come will also do it.

Joy is not to be confused with elation although these feeling states sometimes overlap. Elation is a high that can come and go quickly and is shallower and more transient than joy, which is the gold standard of good human feeling. Joy is a very deeply felt emotion that nourishes and strengthens the self. In hymns and religious writings, it has been located as down in my heart. Simply put, the senses quicken and we feel more alive. The soul is the unit of the mind that monitors the intimate relationship between people and their Maker or Higher Power. Thus when the emotion of joy issues forth, it is already modulated by a fitting degree of humility that makes it more durable and lasting than elation.

One of life's greatest challenges for spiritual exercise is to become able to forgive those who have harmed us in any way. All of us have had experiences that give rise to the thought I'll never be able to forgive someone for this or that. And yet the health of both soul and body requires us to be able to forgive everyone. Many husbands or wives keep a litany of past spousal offenses in the back of their minds for use at the first sign of a recurrent incident, whether real or imagined. Such a list of old grievances could provide a helpful focus for spiritual exercise on days when there are no new candidates for forgiveness. If one has been the victim of a terrible crime the task of forgiveness may seem impossible for a very long time. But God or a Higher Power is present even in criminals and in our worst enemies, and so we must try to love and respect them as fellow human beings. One of the goals of spiritual exercise has to be to enlist the help of God or a Higher Power in overcoming our reluctance to forgive. Forgiving allows us to forget a painful past event and get on with our lives without the recurrent intrusions of physically toxic anger. A powerful amount of prayer may be needed to reach the ideal of forgiveness but prayer for this purpose is an open road to oneness with God, or the fulfillment of our highest ideals.

The soul is a spiritual being that is at once a person, place and thing, encompassing both God and a Higher Power and housing them together with us. It is the most important part of our human nature. The soul permeates our personhood, energizes it and defines it. The soul is who we are, our identity, and how we are, our functions. The soul joins us, in our inner life, with every other human being in the world. We are linked with them by our care and concern and this linkage must be in operation for rationality to survive. As a place, the soul is the tabernacle of God, or a Higher Power. It is a beautiful rendezvous where we can be alone with Both and enjoy the soothing and healing solace of our inner warmth. As a thing, the soul is the entire human body whose maintenance and appropriate upkeep is our personal responsibility. Care of the body is a vital daily task carried out with the soul's approval and increasing our respect for the bodies and personhood of all others.

The soul thrives on our work activities and every job is indeed a vocation, an array of human functions that we carry out for the good of others and for ourselves. The Latin root for the word vocation tells us that it is a calling, with the religious meaning for many of acknowledging God's blessing on our work as a means of doing for others. Hippocrates, in 640 B.C., astutely recognized the role of the physician as an agent of the gods, who bears the same loving responsibility for the care of patients as the gods themselves. He regarded this connection with the deity of his day as a unique badge of honor for his profession. In fact, every profession shares in the distinction of promoting God's or a Higher Power's goals for human betterment. The clergy attend to our spiritual well being, while lawyers pursue the noble goal of equal justice for all. Architects and engineers enhance the beauty of the world and add efficiency to our lives. Accountants and businessmen (and women) monitor the money needed for the charitable aims of the soul, and farmers provide our daily bread. To the extent that these people live by the ideal values of their profession they engage in a daily form of spiritual exercise. By the practice of their profession they profess their faith in God, or in the worth of their highest ideals.

One of the most meaningful and compelling forms of spiritual exercise is the prayer group shared by members of different professions who take a brief weekly time-out from their workday to acknowledge their kinship with one another and with God. They come fresh from their workplace to commune jointly with God and return to it with a greater awareness of God's presence in themselves and others. They bring with them a new perspective on their work, their co-workers and those who will benefit from their work-product. It is a holy perspective that issues forth not only from their own souls but also from the combined energies of the souls of those with whom they are engaged in weekly prayer. Often the participants read a brief passage from scripture that they interpret by pure intuition. This results in the sharing of a considerable number of highly personal and differing meanings. The net result is a significantly enriched understanding of the passage coming from the valuable soul function of intuition.

My favorite experience of spiritual exercise occurs but once a year and yet it yields uplifting memories that continue to nourish the soul for the remainder of the year and a lifetime. It is the annual pilgrimage of the national associations of the Order of Malta from around the world to the shrine of Our Lady of Lourdes. The Knights and Dames of Malta descend on Lourdes, in southern France, during the first week each May, bringing with them some of their poor and desperately ill countrymen in a latter day version of the Great Crusades. The original members of the Order of Malta fought in the war to liberate Jerusalem and The Holy Land in the year 1000 A.D., and then stayed on to care for their own wounded, and sick pilgrims from other parts of the world.

I don't fancy myself a psychohistorian but it seems to me a simple matter of common sense that these men, who had survived a war of bloody hand to hand combat, had to be killers in order to survive. They also must have emerged from it with an overload of the destructive drives that would have made them prime candidates for posttraumatic stress disorders. Their dedication to caring for people who were very sick was a wonderful way to heal an overload of destructive drive energies. The continued and still vigorous life of the Order of Malta, despite many unfavorable moments of near demise in its long history, gives living testimony to the soul-power of its pilgrimages, and dedication to the poor and the sick.

There are three American Associations of the Order: The American in New York, The Federal in Washington, and The Western in San Francisco. Each includes members from around the entire country. For the Washington group, our pilgrimage begins on the last Saturday in January when a team of doctors and nurses from the Order meets with thirty or forty people who have applied to make the trip. Our six doctors and two nurses get well acquainted with every one of them and their companions as well. There is an almost instantaneous bonding that is extremely moving for the participants on both sides. People pour out their hearts and souls about their struggles with cancers and other devastating conditions. Many stand in the very shadow of death, perhaps several months away. Their faith in God and hope for help from Christ's mother, Mary, are inspirational. We feel their pain deeply and are touched by their wonderful hope. A measure of the empathy of our medical staff is the reaction all of us have noticed on arrival home at the end of the day. We peel off our jackets and ties, open our collars, sit back in an easy chair, and just say "WOW!" And then we begin to share this extraordinary day's experience with our spouses. I always feel extremely worn out from exposure to the sadness in our fellow pilgrims' lives, and yet buoyed by their profound hope. Very few expect a total miracle. They are realistic about this possibility, but know they are in need of help and feel confident it will come. I retire early that night to deal with my fatigue, and sleep soundly in anticipation of a productive meeting of the medical staff the next day.

The amount of work that goes into the selection process is something many of our fellow knights and dames are not aware of. Mary Noel Page, our aptly named Chief Nurse, has already spent hours in contact with each potential pilgrim gathering medical and social information and building a rapport that is phenomenal. The meeting gives every one of us a chance to share our observations about the medical condition of our future pilgrims, their illness itself, potential problems on the trip, emotions such as anxiety, depression or anger, and tensions within the family that may be deleterious to health. We have to master these details about everyone we have seen so that we can brief the members of the Order who will look after them on the trip. Most of our members have their own illness or special intentions for the pilgrimage and they share these quite readily. A precious intimacy between the sick and caretakers begins to develop immediately and continues to grow in depth and intensity during the week of the trip. Our members find themselves revealing things about their own childhood, or previous life problems that they never dreamed would become part of the helpful mix of a shared healing togetherness. Our job is to pull the sick in carriages to a range of spiritual events that take place in beautiful surroundings on either side of the Gave River, a powerful stream that surges through the territory of the Shrine. These include Stations of the Cross by the river or on a steep hillside, bathing in springs at the foot of the hillside, a candlelight procession with recitation of the rosary in five languages and outdoor Masses in open tents or at the grotto of the Shrine.

The basic rule of the pilgrimage is that the knights and dames will put the needs and wishes of the sick ahead of their own at all times. This may sound easy, but it is a 24\7 task that requires a great deal of self-vigilance and self-discipline. It is the very essence of the pilgrimage. By concentrating intensely on the value of other human beings, and becoming deeply aware of their struggle with distressing physical disturbances, we are drawn into a special kind of intimacy. We identify with them, become one with them. We share their suffering and they know it. For some, we are standing with them at the very entrance to the Valley of Death, and lending our support to their passage through it. Human nature is a wonderful and privileged state that we can better appreciate when we realize that we are here for the good of one another. This is what the pilgrimage accomplishes for all of us and why we look forward to the opportunity to do it again.

Lourdes is a holy place and the Grotto is at its very heart. It is the site where eighteen meetings took place between Christ's Blessed Mother, Mary, and a peasant girl of Basque extraction named Bernadette Soubirou. The location of these visits is well known because The Blessed Mother asked Bernadette to dig in a barren spot of ground in the

Grotto where she uncovered an underground spring. Bernadette was advised to drink this water, and wash with it, and that it would have a healing effect on those who were sick. These events took place in eighteen fifty-five, and the waters of the Lourdes springs have been used for these purposes ever since. Speaking in the Basque dialect The Blessed Mother identified herself to Bernadette as The Immaculate Conception. Since there was no way that the unlearned Bernadette could have known of this recently promulgated Catholic doctrine it has been cited as evidence for the authenticity of the apparitions.

Immersion in the baths is the absolute high-point of the pilgrimage for most people coming to Lourdes. It is a solemn ritual with two levels of healing: one based on the exchange of warmth with the volunteers who run the bath facilities, and the other a directly spiritual, heart-felt conversation with The Blessed Mother. The baths are housed in male and female pavilions immediately adjacent to the Grotto. Anterooms for undressing accommodate six people at a time, engaged in silent prayer as they disrobe. They are strangers from differing parts of the world but there is a shared feeling of closeness based on anticipation of the very special life experience that lies just ahead. The attendants call us in one at a time to wrap each person in a towel while pilgrims remove their underwear. Immersion at Lourdes recapitulates the primal innocence of the Baptism of our infancy. It takes place in a stone tub filled with fresh spring water like the milieu in the recently reported Baptismal cave of St. John. The water is so sparkling and clear that it is instantly absorbed by the skin, and there is no need for towels to facilitate drying. Many wish to repeat the bath on another day, but even if it only takes place once it becomes a treasured memory for a lifetime.

To apply the concept of The Immaculate Conception to the theme of this book it means that the Blessed Virgin was born without the stain of original sin, and consequently was born without the destructive drives that are at the root of all sin. This would mean that Her Loving and Healing Energies far surpassed those of other human beings, and approached the loving power of an All-Loving God. All of us who have participated in the annual pilgrimages of the Order of Malta are aware that our own supply of healing inner warmth reaches an absolute peak when we are in Lourdes. I suspect this comes about through the on-going spiritual presence of the Blessed Mother at this specially chosen location. I also think it no accident that the Grotto stands in the shadow of the fortress of Lourdes where the destructive drives reigned supreme for centuries in wars between Spain and France.

Do you see miracles in Lourdes? No, but there are some remarkable improvements in health, and some uniquely personal meaningful events. Do you see healing there? Yes, every single day. Very often parents who have had to deal with the daily heartaches of a disabled child develop considerable anger with one another about the best way to treat their ailing youngster. There may be a lot of bickering at the outset of the pilgrimage that quickly gets replaced by handholding and the exchange of loving glances. They emerge from the pilgrimage with a newfound mutual respect. In a similar way people who have been undergoing the self-torture of daily resentment about illness may finally achieve an acceptance of their condition that allows them to experience a rapprochement with God.

The development of healing friendships are a commonplace at Lourdes. My wife and I had such an experience during one of the candle-light processions that we will never forget. It was a rainy night and people were milling around the area in some confusion as we were at the jump-off location. A man with cerebral palsy came along in a motorized wheelchair looking quite distraught. His face was turned in a somewhat upward direction, soaked with rain, and he was obviously lost. We asked if we could help and learned that he was with the French

Association but had become separated from them and couldn't find them. He was sure by now they were already in the procession and he was crying because he had missed his chance to participate. My wife said, in broken French, "Why don't you come with us. Jim and I will stay right with you, we have an extra candle and an umbrella and we'll help you get back to your hotel afterward." He rewarded us with a truly beatific smile, came along and later joined some of the French group on the way home. On the next day we ran into him unexpectedly in front of the baths and he was absolutely beaming. Looking at his twisted body and radiantly beautiful face I felt that I was experiencing the nearness of God. I have had a similar feeling with some of the other crippled humans I have met in Lourdes but never as strongly as with Alexandre. We exchanged name and address cards with him, and he told us that he lives alone in Paris, where he has a few friends who are able to help him. He comes each year to Lourdes with the French Malta group, and we have had a reunion in his hotel or ours every year. He has a severe speech impediment, and speaks only French, but we can always get through to each other as we did on that rainy night.

On the last day of the 2001 pilgrimage we had the kind of extraordinary experience that only occurs in Lourdes. It was a gloomy and rainy day and we decided to light some candles for deceased relatives at the area near the Grotto reserved for that purpose. There was only one other couple there, about our age, and we struck up a conversation with them that quickly became very animated. The husband was British, with an Irish accent acquired from his Irish father. They lived in Scotland and our conversation immediately began to focus on how their parents and grandparents had moved from Ireland to England and then Scotland, whereas ours had involved the migration of great-grandparents from the same part of Ireland to the U.S. I was fascinated with the couple's origins for reasons to be seen. It began to rain more heavily and our conversation had to terminate while our new acquaintances ran for cover and we deployed our umbrella. We had already given our exact home locations for future reference. I lapsed into silence at our parting and my wife said, "You're so silent and you look a little stunned. What's the matter?"

I said, "Do you remember how sad I was that my father had died just before you had a chance to meet him?" She replied, "Yes, of course." "Well," I said, "You've just met my father. I mean if you want to know exactly what he looked like and how he came across to people, you've just seen it. That man was my father's double. It was spooky and sent chills up my spine. I know he wasn't my father but I was asking all those questions to see if they might have been twins. My father was big like he was, same height and even had the same extra weight around the beltline. He had grey-green eyes just like that man and wore the same kind of glasses that made his eyes look large. They had the same high forehead and curly, gray hair and they sounded the same, except my father spoke fast like a New Yorker and didn't have an Irish accent. They even told the same kind of funny stories about themselves. Oh well, I know it wasn't my father but why do things like that happen in Lourdes, and nowhere else in the forty years since my father's death? It gives you a lot to think about, especially if you believe in the migration of the soul after the body's death."

This brings us back to the question of why the pilgrimage is such an effective form of spiritual exercise, and why, indeed, Lourdes has had such a powerful healing effect on human beings. I believe the fundamental therapeutic element is Faith and the fact that God is actually present in every human soul waiting to be actively drawn into our lives. Faith comes first from our parents, then from teachers, and most importantly from one another. When you are with a group of people who have dedicated themselves to helping others, as in a pilgrimage, the

Faith of your fellow pilgrims penetrates your soul and increases its reservoir of Faith, hope and love. In Lourdes you experience the input of Faith from around the entire world. You see it in the faces of the throngs who walk the streets headed for the Grotto. You are inundated by it when you see the stretcher trains pulling into the station from the far reaches of Europe. Jesus Christ stressed the value of Faith in the healing of medical illnesses over and over again, and now there are studies reported in the medical literature that support the beneficial effects of Faith and prayer on serious illness.

My belief that there have been miracles at Lourdes (there are sixty-seven on record) is not simply a matter of Faith. The International Medical Association of Lourdes has established strict medical standards for the evaluation of purported miracles, and they now provide close scrutiny by highly regarded physicians in every specialty. Dr. Alexis Carrell, one of the giants of twentieth century medicine, began a pilgrimage to Lourdes as a miracle skeptic and actually witnessed the miraculous healing of a woman near death from an advanced case of tuberculosis. He described her illness and recovery in his book "A Voyage to Lourdes."

The ultimate goal of spiritual exercise is to create a soul that is so robust, so full of loving energies, that it achieves a permanent modification of the destructive drives and brings us an inner peace. In such a state there is no stranger anxiety. We make our inner warmth available to everyone we meet through a smile and friendly greeting. If they reject us we are moved to compassion instead of anger. We learn to live with our human shortcomings such as impatience, anger, envy or lust and seek to change them through meditation. In this way we can feel the daily presence of an All-Loving God in our lives and turn our flaws into a prayer of thanksgiving that we were born to be caring and rational. We nourish ourselves on all that is beautiful in the world and work to change all that is ugly. Our mission is to develop an inner peace so that all human beings may eventually live in a world at peace.

The human soul is a counterpoise to the destructive drives. The ego and superego are merely tools that aid the soul in keeping the destructive drives in place. God created the human animal with destructive drives to guarantee its survival, but also left a part of His/Her Being within these creatures so they might share their warmth with other people, heal their destructive drives and grow in their capacity to love.

The Soul is an inner storehouse of refined loving energies that is the defining characteristic of human nature. It is a love of the highest quality that survives after death, and continues to serve those who have benefited from it during a lifetime. In life the Soul is our inner warmth, a powerful healing force that can subdue overloads of destructive energies: hatred, anger and even organic illness. God is always within the Soul creating loving relationships that are not self-centered, but exist primarily for the good of the beloved. All human beings deserve our love and respect because they too possess a Soul that harbors an All-Loving God.

Life is a daily pilgrimage, a ceaseless quest for God that finally ends in death and freedom of the Soul to engage its Creator in a new way. Before that time, we search for God in marble temples and humble country churches, in palaces and homeless shelters, until we find God's presence in the inner warmth of our Soul, as a constant, reliable companion, and the Ultimate Source of the power of our love.

About the author

I grew up in a mid-Bronx neighborhood of apartments, and later in the North Bronx, where vacant lots, yards and large frame houses dominated the scene. Stickball was the major sporting pastime in both areas, with the addition of baseball and football in the North. My father owned a diner, and later taverns, and my mother was a former nurse, who was indeed a healer for many of her friends and acquaintances. My four siblings included a brother, five years older, brothers one and four years younger, and a sister, born when I was five. Every summer was spent with our grandparents in Hummelstown, PA, and near-by Hershey. I liked the small town ambience and life much better.

I am indebted to my teachers and supervisors in The Baltimore Psychoanalytic Institute for the durability and enjoyment of my career as a psychiatrist and psychoanalyst. I have no plans to retire for as long as I am physically and mentally able to carry on.

Above all else, my happiness is rooted in my wife, Priscilla, children Maureen, Jimmy and Patrick, daughter-in-law Gabrielle, and grandson Jack. I don't have much free time but can find a few hours each week for some golf, reading and workouts at a fitness center.

Comments on the chapters

Chapter one answers the often asked question about why I pursued a law degree after internship. It details the abuse of patients legally committed to St. Elizabeth's Hospital that I had witnessed while in medical school. The idea of taking a few courses in law school began at that time.I was shocked by conditions there and in my first year of residency at D.C.General I felt a short-fall of good human contact that could be offset by attending night law school. I had no idea that going there would turn out to be a nine year cure.

Chapter two introduces the reader to the cadre of Boston trained physicians who ruled the Department of Internal Medicine at the Georgetown University Hospital. My internship in internal medicine there brought me into intimate contact with all of these doctors, who were healers because of the way they shared their caring energies with patients. Dr. Harold Jeghers was their leader, and he created a Fellowship for me with Dr. Proctor Harvey, Georgetown's renowned cardiologist, to prepare me for my internship. Both of these men shared in the beautiful legacy of Hippocrates, who urged his colleagues to draw on the holiness of their gods in ministering to their patients. I have tried to live up to the high standard of caring set by all three of these physicians. Georgetown's internship was well known for its academic excellence, but an even more important feature was the nurturing provided the interns by department heads and consultants.

Chapter three describes another training program with beneficial consequences to this day. Dr. Grete Bibring, Chief Psychiatrist at Boston's Beth Israel Hospital, was my most important role model for healing. She was one of Freud's most well known trainees, and she told me of his unfulfilled wish to be able to solve the mystery of schizophrenia, in order to enhance our knowledge of human nature. She urged me to take on Freud's quest by taking a position at the D.C.General Hospital where several thousand acutely ill schizophrenics were being admitted each year. The success of our staff in treating them, and the important lessons about human nature that we learned, are the principal "raison d'etre" for this book.

Chapter four describes the plight of an overload of untreatable schizophrenics who were passing through a revolving door at D.C.General on their way to long term incarceration at St. Elizabeth's Hospital.

Chapter five recounts the discovery of the "warming point" in schizophrenia, after three years of failure and frustration in my quest. It was the start of getting through to schizophrenics. My principal task as a teacher had been the making of new admission ward rounds. A burdensome assignment became a gratifying challenge when we learned how to elicit a little bit of warmth in these encounters. There is a conspicuous error in my comment to the resident physicians about Shakespeare being the author of the famous "Hell hath no fury" quotation. It was actually William Congreve's brainchild in the eighteenth century. "Heaven has no rage like love to hatred turned, nor hell a fury like a woman scorned."

Chapter six describes the conquest of violence in our two most dangerous kinds of patients: paranoid schizophrenics who had come to the White House to seek the president's help, and catatonic schizophrenics who were always at risk for violence on a large scale. The healing of Eddie, who was catatonic, convinced us that the sharing of inner warmth could bring about recovery from schizophrenia. Even so, we were just beginning to realize the therapeutic potential of shared warmth.

Chapter seven, about my mother's murder on a quiet Bronx street, was the most difficult one for me to write, but by the time I had it finished I could better appreciate the growth potential in the mourning process. The chancy, and indeed unlikely, way in which I met my future wife strongly suggested that my mother's soul had something to do with it.

Chapter eight gave me a chance to honor my predecessor as Chief Psychiatrist, Dr. Jim Foy. He deserves a major share of the credit for what was accomplished there. I can still remember my shock when he told me of his resignation. I had to grow up quickly for the heavy lifting that was ahead.

Chapters nine and ten really go together as they describe the lead up and final realization of the almost miraculous outcome of our efforts. The site-visits of staff from the Philadelphia General and Bellevue Hospitals was particularly important in establishing credence for the healing of schizophrenics at D.C.G.H. Being a New Yorker myself I was able to enjoy the disbelief of the New York group. We don't want to take a chance on being fooled by anyone. The presence of a healing love drive in everyone was a very important finding.

Chapter eleven, on the discovery of the secrets of human nature promised by Freud, was a very gratifying experience for me. It reminded me of the inner warmth I had shared with Dr. Grete Bibring, and I was certain she would have approved of our discoveries at D.C.General. I considered these as a small token of my appreciation for the rich accumulation of insights she had provided for her staff. Freud's error in his important paper on schizophrenia, "The Case of Schreber" was because he was seeking a sexual explanation for Schreber's psychotic illness when in fact his deep withdrawal was caused by an overload of aggressive urges. The paper is contained in volume twelve of "The Complete Psychological works of Sigmund Freud."

Chapter twelve about Georgetown's withdrawal from D.C.General Psychiatry was another painful one for me to write. I still find it hard to deal with the disillusionment caused by Drs. John Schultz, Murray Grant and the National Institute of Mental Health when they disrupted Georgetown's program at the D.C.G.H.

Chapter thirteen about the successful treatment of a chronic schizophrenic considered unreachable was thought by some of my colleagues to have been a good choice for the opening chapter. This heartwarming case is presented in great detail because it illustrates how effective the sharing of inner warmth can be even for a long-standing and severe chronic schizophrenia. It shatters the myth of untreatable, "process schizophrenia."

Chapter fourteen is one of my favorites because it took me so long to figure out the mechanism by which suicidal depressions were being quickly turned around. I also liked it because it bolstered my belief that the purpose of our existence is simply that we are here for the good of one another.

Chapter fifteen is in there by way of paying tribute to one of my important teachers at Beth Israel, Dr. Arnold Modell. He made life easier for all of us by showing how to deal with patients who come at us with devastating anger.

Chapter sixteen presents the subject of intimacy, a life experience for all of us that highlights the healing value of shared inner warmth. For this reason it is also crucial to Chapter seventeen where Managed Care is taken to task for threatening to abolish the role of shared warmth between doctor and patient. A unique feature of Chapter sixteen is its emphasis on early childhood intimacy outside the family in determining the kind of person we become. In my own case it is clear that early childhood intimacy with Black and Jewish children paved the way for my ease in fitting in with the staffs at D.C.General and the Beth Israel Hospital.

Chapters eighteen, nineteen and twenty depart from the subjects of medical and psychological illness to suggest activities that can provide a high yield of personal growth for all of us. Chapter eighteen deals with the ubiquitous problem of prejudice, nineteen with the value of volunteer activities, and twenty with healing the emotional wounds of the nine/eleven catastrophe.

Chapters twenty-one and twenty-two are the most important ones in the book. They depart from the Twentieth Century, three dimensional model of the mind, (ego, superego and id), to recognize a fourth dimension more powerful by far than the other three. It is the human soul where both God, or a Higher Power, and man, reside and interact. The soul is the organ of the mind that allows us to go beyond our expected human limits, to speed up brain function through intuition, to experience platonic relationships, to appreciate beauty in works of art, music or nature, and to find activities that bring joy, the gold standard of human emotion. Exercises that keep the soul in tip-top shape are the subject of Chapter 22.

Index

www.ingramcontent.com/pod-product-compliance
Lightning Source LLC
Chambersburg PA
CBHW032059280526
45784CB00012B/138